*Individualized Exercise
and
Optimal Physical Fitness*

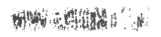

Individualized Exercise
and
Optimal Physical Fitness

A Review Workbook for Men and Women

JOSEPH Di GENNARO, Ed.D.

Department of Health and Physical Education
Herbert H. Lehman College of the City University of New York

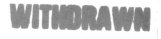
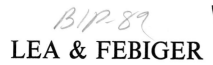

LEA & FEBIGER *Philadelphia · 1974*

Library of Congress Cataloging in Publication Data

Di Gennaro, Joseph.
   Individualized exercise and optimal physical fitness.

   Bibliography: p.
   1. Exercise.   2. Physical fitness.   I. Title.
[DNLM: 1. Gymnastics.   2. Physical fitness.
QT255 D571i 1974]
RA781.D52 1974   613.7   73–9614
ISBN 0–8121–0353–X

Published in Great Britian by Henry Kimpton Publishers, London

PRINTED IN THE UNITED STATES OF AMERICA

To Mom, Dad, Jo, and the Children

There is only one subject matter for education,
and that is life *in* all *its manifestations.*

ALFRED NORTH WHITEHEAD

Preface

Exercise can be a means toward the development of physical fitness, but youngsters and adults should neither have the same fitness expectations nor participate in the same exercises. Individuals differ in many respects, and their fitness goals and physical activity programs should also vary. Regardless of age or sex, one should strive to develop *optimal physical fitness* in line with unique needs. A person is in competition with no one but himself when he attempts to reap physiological and psychological rewards from exercise. Such benefits are assured when an *individualized exercise* program based on realistic goals and personal capacities and interests is carried out with discipline and determination. Thus, within this text there is no attempt to designate a level or degree of physical fitness that should be attained by everyone. Various exercise activities including their strengths and limitations are discussed, but a universal prescription that dictates what kind of exercise to perform and how often to perform it is not presented.

I contend that all persons should become capable of making rational decisions with regard to fitness desires and individualized exercise program design. An understanding of the nature of physical fitness; the physiology of systemic fitness mechanisms; the principles, procedures, and considerations in the construction of exercise programs; and the potential outcomes of regular exercise, which are discussed in this book will provide a basis for such choices. A series of laboratory activities that involve the attainment and analysis of self-descriptive fitness data and provide opportunities to apply learnings in a variety of problem-solving and exercise construction tasks are included.

Because of the rather in-depth study of exercise and fitness, the text is most appropriate for use in the educational setting. However, a comprehension of the material presented and the successful completion of laboratory activities should assure a more rational approach to fitness and exercise, in which decisions and judgments are based on the knowledge of exercise rather than on propaganda or whim. Lastly, I hope that the book will contribute to the reader's desire and ability to exercise and evaluate physical fitness effectively throughout life. These desires seem to be of special significance, because we live in an era when many negative social forces promote inactivity and a lack of concern for physical health, especially among the urban and suburban masses in America.

New York, New York   JOSEPH DI GENNARO

Contents

Individualized Exercise
and
Optimal Physical Fitness

CHAPTER ONE

The Nature of Physical Fitness

. . . The Greeks knew that intelligence and skill can only function at the peak of their capacity when the body is healthy and strong; that hardy spirits and tough minds usually inhabit sound bodies. In this sense, physical fitness is the basis of all activities in our society, and if our bodies grow soft and inactive, if we fail to encourage physical development and prowess, we will undermine our capacity for thought, for work and for the use of those skills vital to an expanding and complex America.

JOHN F. KENNEDY

There has been a resurgence of interest in and concern for physical fitness since the 1950s. Fitness levels of children in the United States and other nations have been compared. Early in his administration President Kennedy delegated to a special White House Committee on Health and Fitness the responsibility "to formulate and carry out a program to improve the physical condition of the nation."[11] Educators[9,10] have theorized that physical fitness is an integral component of health. Others are more skeptical. They have challenged the emphasis given to physical fitness, because they believe that the framework and meaning of the concept are not universally accepted. A celebrated argument of critics is that one can fail a physical fitness test and yet easily meet the physiological requirements of everyday life.

It is intellectually immature to negate the educational worth of this subject matter because it is neither totally understood nor universal in conceptualization. The fact that wide spheres of the unknown exist for all sciences and social sciences does not negate the significance of what is known. A completely objective and acceptable concept of human health may not exist, for health ideas and practices are continually being revised in light of

1

scientific discovery.   Yet, an intelligent person values optimal health and strives to attain it through the utilization of the most advanced knowledge in health science.

Despite an abundance of leisure and a general acceptance of the idea that physical fitness is desirable and that exercise is probably beneficial, regular physical activity is placed quite low on the list of priorities of most Americans. When one observes protruding mid-sections and fat, fleshy limbs; hears reports of aching muscles and sore backs following minimal muscular stress, and of breathlessness, discomfort, and nausea when the heart and lungs are taxed; and knows the number of orthopedic disorders associated with weakened muscles and joints, it becomes evident that the physical fitness of many people, including our younger generation, is slowly becoming horrendous.[18]

Those who value fitness often approach exercise unscientifically.   Consider the searchers of "instant fitness"!   They invest time and money in vibrating machines, exercise wheels, inflatable waist and limb belts, weight-reducing pills, and countless other unproved products and schemes claimed by manufacturers to strengthen muscles, firm mid-sections, increase body stamina, and reduce body fat without sweat, toil, or discomfort.   The realization that choices concerning the kinds, amounts, and purposes of exercise cannot be made effectively supports the contention that knowledge of *individualized exercise and optimal physical fitness* is relatively lacking.   Not too long ago the "Charles Atlas" build was the symbol of physical fitness. Today it is clear that being physically fit involves much more than being a muscle man.   One must be a student of exercise and fitness if he is to make exercise participation a constructive and productive health measure.

THE HUMAN MACHINE*

What a piece of machinery the human body really is!   It is intricately constructed and capable of operating with greater efficiency, lower cost, and less wear and tear than most man-made machines.   Had it been built to use common fuel, the human machine could sustain life for 10 days on just 1 gallon of motor oil.

More than 6,000 quarts of blood can be ejected daily by the heart, which is a tremendous accomplishment because the body contains only 4 to 6 quarts of blood.   Even during sleep this miraculous pump continues to supply life-sustaining blood to every body cell.

Skeletal muscle, varying in size and shape, constitutes a natural human motor system.   Muscle tissue, 75% of which is water, has a pulling capacity of 140 pounds per square inch of cross section.   About 400 billion cylindrical muscle cells averaging 1/600 inch in diameter provide the energy that sets the skeletal levers of the machine into a variety of movements.   Human bone,

* The concept of the "Human Machine" was presented by Arthur Steinhaus,[14] and many of the facts discussed in this monograph are condensed from his work.

which has twice the strength of oakwood, can resist loads of 2 tons per square inch.

The nervous system, the electrical wiring system that triggers all human function, is composed of billions of nerve strands varying in length from a fraction of an inch to 6 feet. The nervous system's pathways and functioning mechanisms are so complex that they still baffle scientists. It has been theorized that a computer equal in operation to the human brain, which alone contains approximately 10 billion nerve cells, would occupy a space comparable to that of a city skyscraper.

MUSCLE ACTIVATION AND METABOLISM

The trillions of cells in the body are in constant need of nourishment for continual growth, repair, and functioning. The supply of nutritional materials and the removal of wastes through circulatory mechanisms permit *homeostasis*, the biochemical balance within the body cells that allows their uninterrupted operation. The total of all the biochemical reactions resulting in fuel utilization and heat and waste production is called *metabolism*.

Skeletal muscle is the body's largest organ accounting for as much as 40 to 60% of total body weight. The rate of metabolism within activated muscle tissue may be 100 times that of the resting level.[3] Thus, the highest metabolic rate of which the body is capable occurs during the performance of strenuous muscular work. Water and foods processed by the digestive system are replenished periodically by eating and drinking. But the human machine is not capable of storing oxygen despite the on-going consumption of this valuable element by cells. Vital organs, including the heart and brain, are incapable of life and function if adequate oxygen is not continually supplied. Oxygen is used by muscle tissue to ward off the buildup of *lactic acid*, an end product of metabolism proportional to muscle activation. Its continued accumulation results in reduced muscle response.

The red blood cells (*erythrocytes*) contain a protein called *hemoglobin* (Hb). It combines with oxygen (O_2), diffused into the blood stream of the lungs from inhaled air, to form *oxyhemoglobin* (HbO_2) which is carried to the cells. Hemoglobin also combines with carbon dioxide (CO_2), transporting this end product of metabolism from local tissues through the blood to the lungs for expiration from the body. Women have about a 10% lower concentration of hemoglobin in the blood than do men. Because of this, as well as other structural and functional factors, females have a lower potential to attain and sustain high degrees of metabolism resulting from muscular work (see Chapter Six).

MUSCULAR WORK CAPACITY

The amount of positive work accomplished is determined by calculating the distance a force or resistance is moved ($W = F \times D$, where W is work accomplished, F is force, and D is distance). Muscular work is often mea-

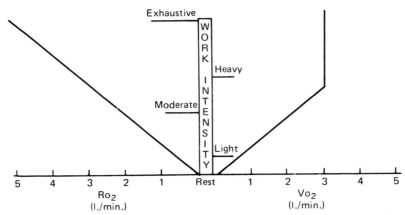

FIGURE 1.1. Ro_2 and Vo_2 in response to muscular work intensity. Ro_2 continues to rise linearly with an increase in work intensity, but Vo_2 remains the same (3 l. O_2/min.) when a certain work intensity level is reached.

sured in the exercise performance laboratory in kilopond meters (kpm) or foot-pounds. *

Work intensity is the amount of work performed per unit of time. The number of foot-pounds or kilopond meters accomplished can be increased by increasing either the work load or the rate of performance. For example, a simple performance work task, such as running a mile, can be intensified by running faster (rate) or by wearing a 10-pound belt (load).

Naturally, the longer the duration of muscular work at a specified intensity, the more work accomplished. Thus, running 10 miles per hour for six minutes produces twice the number of foot-pounds of work as does running at the same speed for three minutes. Usually the less intense the muscular work, the longer it can be sustained. Rest periods reduce the effects of high intensity work by providing muscles (also heart and lungs) an opportunity to be replenished with needed fuels and oxygen. Research findings seem to indicate that *intermittent work*, that is, alternating periods of work (5 to 30 seconds) with equal periods of rest, is the most effective and least stressful method of handling moderate to heavy muscular activity.[4] Thus, strenuous activities, such as housework, waxing a car, gardening, and shoveling snow, might be performed more safely and efficiently when brief work bouts are alternated with rest periods.

The demands for oxygen by working muscle tissues or the *O_2 requirement* (Ro_2) and the volume of oxygen consumed or the *O_2 consumption* (Vo_2) are proportional to work intensity† (Figure 1.1). The higher the Vo_2 the more readily the Ro_2 can be satisfied.

* One kilopond meter is the force acting on the mass of 1 kg. at normal acceleration of gravity. One foot-pound equals 3.2389×10^{-4} kcal. A 150-pound person who walks or jogs 900 feet has performed 135,000 foot-pounds of work (150×900).

† The consumption of 1 liter of oxygen involves the burning of 5 calories. One calorie equals 3087 foot-pounds or 426 kpm.

When the Ro_2 of sustained muscular work does not exceed the Vo_2, the individual is performing at a *"steady state"* or *aerobically* (has adequate free oxygen to sustain the activity), and there is no significant accumulation of lactic acid. The highest Vo_2 level that can be attained during aerobic work (the highest steady state that can be reached) is called *maximal aerobic capacity*. During work without adequate free oxygen or *anaerobic work*, the Ro_2 exceeds the Vo_2 resulting in an *oxygen debt* buildup. The more intense the muscular work, the quicker the debt accumulation (Figure 1.2).

Foods utilized in muscular work are carbohydrates (glucose and glycogen) and fats (free fatty acids). During short efforts, anaerobic processes, involving the burning of carbohydrates, assume a dominant role; whereas the utilization of free fatty acids takes place during prolonged periods of aerobic work.[4]

The capacity to persist in anaerobic work or the O_2 *debt tolerance* is determined by physiological and psychological variables (e.g., lactic acid buildup and endurance of pain and discomfort). A person cannot run full speed for as long a time as he can jog (aerobic task), because sprinting involves a rapid O_2 debt buildup beyond the level of individual tolerance. That high O_2 debt tolerance and Vo_2 capacities enhance the potential for moderate anaerobic work is evidenced by the work capacity formula:[16]

$$\text{Muscular Work Capacity (min.)} = \frac{O_2 \text{ debt tolerance (l.)}}{Ro_2 \text{ (l./min.)} - Vo_2 \text{ (l./min.)}}$$

Naturally, the oxygen debt is repaid to muscle, heart, and lung tissues, following the cessation of work, through the continuous functioning of oxygen transport mechanisms.

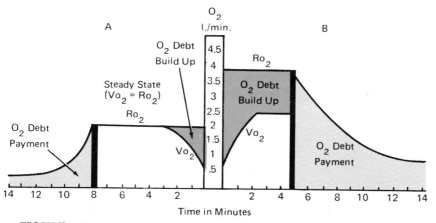

FIGURE 1.2. Aerobic and anaerobic work. A, During aerobic work there is minimal O_2 debt buildup that ceases when Vo_2 equals Ro_2. O_2 debt payment takes place quite quickly (as compared to a large O_2 debt buildup). B, This work task is anaerobic because the maximal aerobic capacity of the performer is not sufficient to meet the Ro_2 of the task. It cannot be performed for more than five minutes and O_2 debt payment will involve a considerable period of time.

PHYSICAL FITNESS AND MUSCULAR WORK

Exercise physiologists contend that maximal aerobic capacity is a measure of muscular work capacity.[4] Maximal Vo_2 can be evaluated through the use of three muscular work devices: the motor driven treadmill, the bicycle ergometer, and the step-up bench (Figure 1.3). The amount of work performed during tests can be controlled and calculated with these pieces of equipment.

Heart rate (HR), the number of heart beats per minute, is the major criterion of Vo_2. With certain exceptions, during muscular work heart rate is directly proportional to Vo_2 in normal individuals. The lower the increment in heart rate during muscular activity, the greater the Vo_2 (see Chapter Three). Heart rate is also a valid indicator of work intensity. Table 1.1 shows approximate figures for Vo_2, heart rate, and caloric expenditure of various exercise activities in a moderately fit person. The exact stress an exercise or work task produces depends on the individual's muscular work capacity or physical fitness level. Running 2 miles in 14 minutes would probably exhaust an average male but not even tax Jim Ryun, the premier distance runner. Chris Evert, a highly fit female, engages regularly in sustained tennis practice that would produce fatigue in a sedentary woman.

Both the requirement for and consumption of oxygen during muscular work greatly depend on three components of physical fitness: *lean body weight, neuromuscular efficiency,* and *cardiovascular-respiratory efficiency.* Fat or *adipose* tissue is inert. It intensifies the oxygen demand and energy cost of

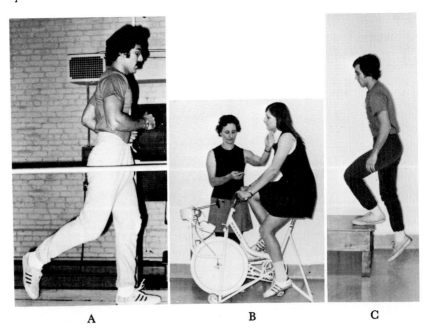

FIGURE 1.3. Performance of work in the Exercise Performance Laboratory.
A, Treadmill; B, bicycle ergometer; C, step-up bench.

TABLE 1.1
O$_2$ Consumption, Heart Rate, and Caloric Expenditure
for Typical Recreational Exercise Activities in
a Moderately Fit Person

Exercise Activity	Classification of Intensity	V$_{O_2}$	Heart Rate	Calories per Minute
Baseball Ping-Pong Volleyball	Very light to light	0.4–1	80–99	2–5
Calisthenics Dancing Golf Tennis	Moderate	1–1.5	100–119	5–7.5
Cycling Handball Jogging Squash Swimming	Heavy to unduly heavy	1.5–3	120–179	7.5–15
Sprinting Skiing	Exhaustive	3	180	15

muscular work without providing a proportional increase in oxygen delivery. Excessive fat burdens body organs including the heart, because fat must be furnished with blood. The reduction of adipose tissue lessens the metabolic costs of physical activity and modifies stress to the heart, lungs, blood vessels, muscles, and joints.

Neuromuscular efficiency means that the muscles and joints, the blood vessels that supply them, and the nerves that innervate them are healthy and fit. Muscle strength and endurance and joint flexibility and stability are characteristics of an effective neuromuscular system.

Cardiovascular-respiratory efficiency, sometimes called endurance, stamina, or wind, depends on the functioning of the lungs, heart, blood vessels, and blood, which operate as a unit in ingesting and transporting oxygen to muscle tissues where it is consumed. For this reason, these organs will be referred to as the *O$_2$ transport system.* Any pulmonary, cardiac, or muscle-joint weakness limits the human machine's ability to attain, sustain, and recover from heightened levels of work metabolism. When the physiological condition of these organs is improved, maximal aerobic capacity and the ability to perform maximal and submaximal muscular work with lower energy costs are enhanced. Since performance of muscular work in part reflects the health of the heart and blood vessels, tests of work capacity have been utilized in the diagnosis and treatment of cardiovascular diseases.

A REALISTIC PHYSICAL FITNESS MODEL

Physical fitness is influenced by age, sex, constitutional makeup, and mode of life. The "blue print" for physical health and fitness is supplied by heredity. In biological terms, the human body as it appears (*phenotype*) is an expression of the organism as the genes alone would determine it to be (*genotype*). Every male and female begin life with a morphological and functional potential, which sets limits for health and physical fitness.[9] Body

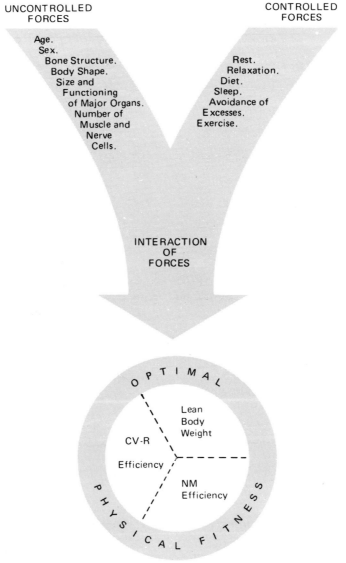

FIGURE 1.4. Schematic representation of optimal physical fitness.

shape; proneness to obesity; bone structure; size and condition of the heart, lungs, and visceral organs; and total number of muscle and nerve cells within the body are fixed at birth. Some persons are born with a high potential for physical fitness and work performance while others are not. It is not within man's power to control these constitutional variables. However, even a poor endowment does not imply that one should be fatalistic and regard any effort to enhance fitness as futile. Total life style, including diet, relaxation, sleep, avoidance of excesses, and participation in appropriate kinds and amounts of exercise, can offset natural forces that contribute to excessive body fat, an inefficient O_2 transport system, and neuromuscular weaknesses. Astrand[4] believes that the dimensions and functions for maximal aerobic capacity can be favorably influenced by exercise during childhood and teenage years when growth and development take place. Constructive health measures cannot cancel genetic limitations, but they can aid the development of *optimal physical fitness* (Figure 1.4), the maximal fitness level predetermined by genotype. A mode of living characterized by infrequent exercise, overeating, and destructive health habits, such as the excessive consumption of alcohol or drugs, can gradually reduce each component of fitness to a subminimal level even when positive constitutional forces exist.

Acceptance of the reality that hereditary and environmental factors predispose twentieth-century men to decreased fitness levels reinforces the significance of the value of exercise and participation in proper physical activity. Truth, knowledge, and constructive action are man's allies in his battle to modify his nature favorably.

EXERCISE AND FITNESS MISCONCEPTIONS

Outstanding amateur and professional athletic achievement does not reflect the level of fitness or exercise participation among average individuals. Most sport enthusiasts are spectators, and little physiological benefit is derived by viewing the athletic feats of others.

An athlete in a state of optimal physical fitness is prepared for the obstacles and stresses of sport. However, an individual can be quite fit though poorly skilled in many sports (Table 1.2).

Some people mistakenly contend that physical activity is for the athlete or "superfit" person. They believe that unfit persons leading sedentary lives should refrain from exercise. Others are of the opinion that strenuous physical activity is for men not women. Such viewpoints and judgments lack rationality and logic. Prior to the technological age muscular work was a necessity for all Americans, including women.

A male or female is neither too sedentary nor too old to derive positive rewards from individualized exercise. The consensus of physicians and physiologists is that the body should be taxed regularly with muscular work if it is to operate efficiently at rest and during periods of stress. Of course, one should abide by the principles of training, and gear exercise toward

TABLE 1.2
Physical Fitness Components and Athletic Performance Variables

Physical Fitness Components	Athletic Performance Variables*
Lean body weight: body state without excessive adipose tissue Cardiovascular-respiratory efficiency: capacity of heart, blood vessels, and lungs to deliver oxygen to body tissues Neuromuscular efficiency: muscular strength and endurance and joint strength and flexibility (capacity to move through full range of motion)	Anticipation: ability to make judgments or to perceive events early Balance: ability to maintain equilibrium in a fixed or moving position Coordination: smooth or graceful flow of movement Agility: ability of whole body or body parts to change direction rapidly Reaction time: ability to react to a stimulus quickly Speed: movement of total body from one place to another in short period of time Physical fitness: lean body weight, cardiovascular-respiratory efficiency, and neuromuscular efficiency

*These are some of the motor variables requisite to successful athletic performance. They are specific to the nature of the sport, and some are more crucial than others, depending on the particular sport.

realistic goals (see Chapter Six). Striving to attain a degree of fitness beyond the limits set by constitutional makeup, age, and sex is frustrating and can be detrimental to health.

The beneficial outcomes of exercise are reaped during one's active days. There is no justification for discontinuing physical activity on the grounds that benefits derived in the past will carry over to the future. The human machine, designed for movement and work, becomes less effective with inaction than action. As muscle activity dwindles, inevitable consequences occur—a reduced capacity for work; lowered levels of functioning in heart, lungs, blood vessels, muscles, bones and joints; and an increased potential for accumulation of adipose tissue. Contrary to a persistent American philosophy, it also appears that the so-called "good life" may, in fact, be the unhealthy life, perhaps even the shortened life (see Chapter Seven). Prior to a discussion of the resultants of inactivity and activity it should be worthwhile to study each component of fitness in detail and to determine the proper methods of developing optimal physical fitness.

REFERENCES

1. Adams, William C., et al. *Foundations of Physical Activity*. Champaign, Ill.: Stipes Publishing Company, 1968.
2. American Medical Association. *The Wonderful Human Machine*. Chicago: American Medical Association, 1961.
3. Andersen, K. L. The Cardiovascular System in Exercise. In H. B. Falls (Editor), *Exercise Physiology*. New York: The Academic Press, 1968.

4. Astrand, L., and K. Rodahl. *Textbook of Work Physiology.* New York: McGraw-Hill Book Company, 1970.
5. Buskirk, Elsworth. An Introduction to Exercise and Performance Evaluation. Proceedings of the National Workshop on Exercise in the Prevention, in the Evaluation, and in the Treatment of Heart Disease. (Supplement to the *Journal of the South Carolina Medical Association*), December, 1969.
6. Corbin, Charles B., et al. *Concepts in Physical Education With Laboratories and Experiments.* Dubuque, Iowa: Wm. C. Brown Co., Publishers, 1970.
7. Falls, Harold. The Relative Energy Requirements of Various Physical Activities in Relation to Physiological Strain. Proceedings of the National Workshop on Exercise in the Prevention, in the Evaluation, and in the Treatment of Heart Disease. (Supplement to the *Journal of the South Carolina Medical Association*), December, 1969.
8. Giese, Warren. Exercise Programs: Types, Directions and Dangers. Proceedings of the National Workshop on Exercise in the Prevention, in the Evaluation, and in the Treatment of Heart Disease. (Supplement to the *Journal of the South Carolina Medical Association*), December, 1969.
9. Hoyman, Howard S. Our Modern Concept of Health. In J. H. Humphrey, et al. (Editors), *Readings in Health Education.* Dubuque, Iowa: Wm. C. Brown Co., Publishers, 1964.
10. Johnson, Perry B., et al. *Physical Education: A Problem-Solving Approach to Health and Fitness.* New York: Holt, Rinehart & Winston, 1966.
11. Kennedy, John F. The Soft American. *Sports Illustrated*, 13:15–23, 1960.
12. Kraus, H., and W. Raab. *Hypokinetic Disease.* Springfield, Ill.: Charles C Thomas, Publishers, 1961.
13. Ricci, Benjamin. *Physical and Physiological Conditioning for Men.* Dubuque, Iowa: Wm. C. Brown Co., Publishers, 1966.
14. Steinhaus, A. H. *Toward an Understanding of Health and Physical Education.* Dubuque, Iowa: Wm. C. Brown Co., Publishers, 1963.
15. Taylor, H. L. Exercise and Metabolism. In W. Johnson (Editor), *Science and Medicine of Exercise and Sports.* New York: Harper & Row, Publishers, 1960.
16. Updyke, W., and P. Johnson. *Principles of Modern Physical Education, Health and Recreation.* New York: Holt, Rinehart & Winston, 1970.
17. Van Huss, Wayne, et al. *Physical Activity in Modern Living.* Englewood Cliffs, N.J.: Prentice-Hall, Inc., 1960.
18. York, Tom. Who Buys Physical Education. Speech delivered to National Convention of American Association of Health, Physical Education and Recreation. Cobo Hall, Detroit, Mich., April 3, 1971.

CHAPTER TWO

Obesity and Its Control

For we, in this generation and in the United States, are the pampered of our planet. . . . We are the fat of the land: never in history, nowhere else in the world have such numbers of human beings eaten so much, exerted themselves so little, and become and remained so fat. We have come suddenly into the land of milk and honey, and we look it. And we suffer because of it.

JEAN MAYER

Abnormalities in body weight limit the performance of stressful muscular work. *Obesity*, the condition in which the body is loaded with extra weight of adipose tissue, hinders the functioning of the organs utilized in muscular work more than does excessive thinness. A minimum amount of adipose tissue is deemed necessary for body insulation, prevention of infection, and storage of reserve energy; but fat in excess of *14%* of the body mass for males and *20%* for females, regardless of age, is indicative of obesity.[8] Fat accumulates in subcutaneous areas, that is, just beneath the skin, and in and around the heart, muscles, and viscera (body organs), causing enlargement and reduced functioning. (From a review of the literature, a recommended minimum amount of body fat could not be discovered.)

Obese people often lack grace, agility, and other motor requisites to efficient movement. Their inability to sustain demanding athletic, household, and everyday work tasks is due to the burden of supporting and transporting a heavier body mass, heightened metabolic requirements of muscle activity, and reduced cardiovascular-respiratory and neuromuscular functioning levels created by the stores of internal and external fatty tissue. Based on the physiology and psychology of obesity it appears that movement inability combined with poor muscular work capacity magnifies obesity problems (Figure 2.1).

Obesity can be considered a health hazard for men and women, because it is associated with both a higher incidence of several degenerative diseases

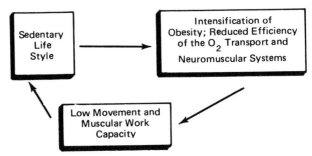

FIGURE 2.1. The obesity cycle. Inability to perform and endure in muscular work often leads the obese person to choose a sedentary life style. Prolonged muscular inactivity can intensify obesity and the accompanying O_2 transport and neuromuscular weaknesses, further reducing work capacity.

and a reduction in life expectancy (see Chapter Seven). Yet, a great number of Americans will join the ranks of the obese unless ameliorative steps are initiated to offset conditions producing fatness.

ETIOLOGY OF OBESITY

The energy values of foods and the rate of heat energy utilized in the metabolic processes are expressed in calories.* The rate of energy expended during internal operations of the body at rest (heart rate, respiration, activity in alimentary canal, and tonus of skeletal muscle) is the *basal metabolic rate* (BMR).† Metabolic rate and caloric expenditure increase as internal body activities heighten.

In order to maintain a daily *caloric* or *energy balance*, the caloric intake from food must equal the caloric output. A caloric intake greater than output due to overeating, underactivity, or both is termed a *positive caloric balance*. Unutilized digested foods are broken down and stored within the body predominantly in the form of adipose tissue.

Degree and type of obesity are highly dependent on causation. It is seldom possible to diagnose with certainty the exact disturbances through which the individual becomes and remains obese. Biometric regulatory mechanisms within the brain and local body tissues tend to balance daily food ingestion in accordance with energy needs. If the *biometric regulation* fails over an extended time, the resulting caloric imbalance causes a weight gain or loss. Impairment to the food intake center in the brain that regulates appetite (the desire for food) can cause habitual overeating. Malfunctions within local body cells can also produce overeating, or the accumulation of

* A calorie is the amount of energy required to raise the temperature of 1 kilogram of water 1 degree centigrade.
† The basal metabolic rates for a 160-pound male and 120-pound female are approximately 76 and 58 calories per hour, respectively.

fat in the absence of overeating. Biometric regulatory disturbances at brain and local levels can be attributed, at times, to shifts in hormone concentrations within the body.[11] Because no biological phenomenon is completely independent of genetic direction, a predisposition to some forms of obesity is also a reality. Excessive eating and inactivity, like other choices of man, are in certain cases psycho-emotional responses, compensations for tensions, frustration, fear, anxiety, and withdrawal.

In sum, it is difficult to draw qualitative conclusions with regard to the etiology of obesity, because each problem is complex and unique. It appears that for twentieth-century man a host of interacting physiological, psychological, and sociocultural factors set the stage for obesity, or, at least, the potentialities for overeating and sedentary living. This conclusion in no way detracts from the physiological reality that a consistent daily positive caloric balance is, for the most part, requisite to significant accumulations of adipose tissue.

CREEPING OBESITY

Creeping obesity is the term applied to the modern-day fatness producer and involves the gradual accretion of adipose tissue beginning in the late college and early adult years. Food intake is usually not curbed in proportion to the decline in caloric expenditure which accompanies the inactive living style often assumed after reaching the twenties and thirties. As a matter of fact, caloric intake actually increases in response to sedentary living habits.[11]

Even if approximately the same body weight were maintained, active tissue is progressively replaced by adipose tissue as one ages. Therefore, those with large body frames or physiques are naturally prone to obesity. The gradual drop in basal metabolic rate occurring automatically with chronological aging (holding all other variables constant) could account for a 12-pound increase between the ages of 25 and 30 years.[12] Thus, even when a program of weight control is initiated, there is no guarantee that creeping obesity will be competely ameliorated.

APPRAISING OBESITY AND THINNESS

A perfectly valid and objective tool for evaluating degree of thinness or of obesity does not exist. Body type, total body weight, and percent of body fat are three criteria used in determining body weight abnormality. One should comprehend the nature of the information derived through these measures.

Body type is a categorical classification of the human anatomy based on shape, structure, and relative predominance of bone, muscle, and adipose tissue. The three body classifications are *endomorph*, *mesomorph*, and *ectomorph* (Figure 2.2). An appraisal of body type can be made by viewing front, back, and profile full-length standing positions and judging the firmness of the muscles of the extremities and mid-section by touch. The degree to which the body features meet endomorphic, mesomorphic, and ectomorphic

MALE

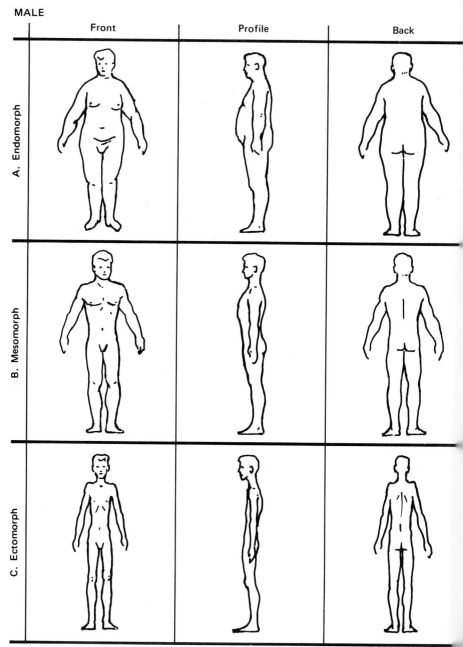

FIGURE 2.2. Major body types. A, Endomorph: oval-shaped person with concentration of weight in the center of the body, abdominal sag, flabby limbs, and poorly toned muscles. B, Mesomorph: husky, big chested person endowed with dense muscles and huge, strong bones. Although the body mass is well proportioned,

FEMALE

Front	Profile	Back	
			A. Endomorph
			B. Mesomorph
			C. Ectomorph

this body type has a tendency to accumulate adipose tissue in later adult years, especially if inactive. C, Ectomorph: extreme thinness, protruding neck, sunken chest, round shoulders, undersized musculature, and a fragile skeletal system characterize this body type.

characteristics is subjectively rated on a scale ranging from 1 to 7. The more the anatomy meets the body type criteria, the higher the point value. The numerical description of body type includes a rating for each classification. A 6-4-2 arrangement would be indicative of high endomorphy, average mesomorphy, and low ectomorphy.

Body type evaluations provide little objective information relating to fatness. Despite the fact that most endomorphs range from extreme to near obesity, some of those rated low on the scale may be below the 14% fat level. Although it appears that nature would be intolerant of obesity in the ectomorph, the possibility does exist.

The comparison of total body weight in pounds to ideal weight provides an objective underweight-overweight measure. Ideal weights are based on the averages of total body pounds for individuals of a similar height, age, and sex. Faulty procedures utilized in the construction of ideal weight tables, including the lack of systematic control of subject's body frame and clothing variables, threaten the validity of the average weights calculated. In recent tables formulated according to varying body frames, there was a failure to incorporate a set criterion for body frame classification. Table 2.1 gives desirable weights for men and women 25 years of age and older.

Obesity is not quite the same as overweight. Correlation figures for total body weight and subcutaneous fat measures reported in scientific studies are positive but not consistently high.[11] A person can weigh more than his ideal weight without being obese (and vice versa). Lean mesomorphs are often overweight due to large, heavy, functional skeletal muscle structures rather than excess fat.

Overweight indices are not as valuable as subcutaneous body fat measures obtained with an instrument known as a skinfold caliper. Percent of body fat, the most valid criterion for evaluation of obesity, can be estimated by obtaining skinfold thickness measures.* The measurement is taken by pinching a full fold of skin and subcutaneous tissue between the thumb and forefinger of the left hand. The fold is held firmly and pulled away from underlying muscle. The subject should flex the muscle briefly, after the tester pinches the fold, to avoid grasping muscle tissue. The caliper is applied to the fold about 1 centimeter below the fingers. Thus the pressure on the fold at the point measured is exerted by the caliper and not by the fingers. When the handle is released, permitting the full force of caliper-arm pressure, the dial is read to the nearest millimeter (Figure 2.3).

OBESITY PANACEAS

A universal treatment for obesity that is completely safe, permanent, and effective does not exist. Delicate problems probably require the professional services of physicians, psychologists, and nutritionists. Americans who de-

---

* Percent of body fat is determined precisely through underwater weighing which is an intricate laboratory procedure. Correlation figures for underwater weighing and subcutaneous skinfold measures of body fat have been positive.

TABLE 2.1.
Metropolitan Life Insurance Co. Tables of Desirable
Weights† (in Pounds) for Men and Women of
Ages 25 * and Over (Indoor Clothing)

Men			
Height (with shoes on— 1″ heels) Feet Inches	Small Frame	Medium Frame	Large Frame
5 2	112–120	118–129	126–141
5 3	115–123	121–133	129–144
5 4	118–126	124–136	132–148
5 5	121–129	127–139	135–152
5 6	124–133	130–143	138–156
5 7	128–137	134–147	142–161
5 8	132–141	138–152	147–166
5 9	136–145	142–156	151–170
5 10	140–150	146–160	155–174
5 11	144–154	150–165	159–179
6 0	148–158	154–170	164–184
6 1	152–162	158–175	168–189
6 2	156–167	162–180	173–194
6 3	160–171	167–185	178–199
6 4	164–175	172–190	182–204

Women			
Height (with shoes on— 2″ heels) Feet Inches	Small Frame	Medium Frame	Large Frame
4 10	92– 98	96–107	104–119
4 11	94–101	98–110	106–122
5 0	96–104	101–113	109–125
5 1	99–107	104–116	112–128
5 2	102–110	107–119	115–131
5 3	105–113	110–122	118–134
5 4	108–116	113–126	121–138
5 5	111–119	116–130	125–142
5 6	114–123	120–135	129–146
5 7	118–127	124–139	133–150
5 8	122–131	128–143	137–154
5 9	126–135	132–147	141–158
5 10	130–140	136–151	145–163
5 11	134–144	140–155	149–168
6 0	138–148	144–159	153–173

* For those between 18 and 25, subtract 1 pound for each year under 25.
† Courtesy of the Metropolitan Life Insurance Company.

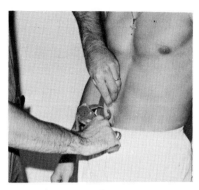
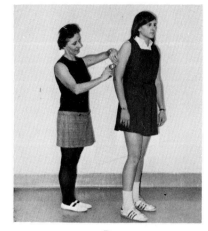

A   B

FIGURE 2.3. Skinfold measurements determined with a caliper. A, Abdominal skinfold being measured in young man. B, Triceps skinfold being measured in female student.

sire the quick, easy remedy spend millions of dollars a year on reducing cocktails, miracle foods, diet pills, slenderizing belts, starvation diets, and a host of other obesity cure-alls. Many popular weight reduction programs involve questionable procedures that are sometimes agonizing and potentially hazardous to health.

Diets that prescribe a drastic curtailment in daily caloric intake of 1000 or more calories may lessen resistance to infection, cause anemia, and produce a higher-than-normal blood uric acid level. Daily fasting, except for the ingestion of one large meal, can provoke digestive and metabolic disturbances. The complex, unpleasant sensation of hunger resulting from strict periodic starvation and liquid dieting has been known to produce tension, anxiety, dizziness, and sleeplessness.[8] Starvation is not a sound way to eliminate stores of body fat, because protein as well as adipose tissue may be used as a source of energy in maintaining internal metabolic activity during periods of extreme food deprivation.

Any diet that involves the complete avoidance of a whole food class, such as fats, is unsound nutritionally, and is not a guaranteed deterrent to a gain in body fat. Carbohydrates, fat, and protein (the three basic foodstuffs) have a common pathway in the final stages of their metabolic breakdown. Fat from excessive carbohydrate and protein is synthetized in the liver and transported to fat cells. Thus, when enough calories from any of the basic foodstuffs are consumed to create a positive caloric balance, a rise in body fat can be expected.[5] The most valid criticism of the starvation-type diet is its lack of permanency in battling obesity. Once it is discontinued and regular eating habits are resumed, weight is slowly gained.

There is a lucrative commercial market for pills that curb the appetite. However, such pills are expensive and contain amphetamine, a stimulant-type drug which can produce hyperactivity as well as other unhealthy side effects. When reduction takes place, adipose tissue seems to be removed from body areas with highest fat concentration. Thus, the fat reduction benefits manufacturers claim for "spot reducing" devices, such as vibrators and inflatable waist and limb belts, seem highly exaggerated. A steam or sauna bath can cause weight reductions, because body fluids are eliminated through excessive sweating. However, such weight is usually regained just as quickly as it is lost when liquids are taken to maintain a safe internal water balance.

EFFECTIVE OBESITY CONTROL

Persons with slight to moderate obesity and others prone to creeping obesity can undertake ameliorative actions that are healthful and permanently effective. The consensus of authorities is that a combination program of regular exercise and slight curtailment of food intake can be a reasonably efficient obesity control procedure. The expenditure of more calories each day than one ingests results in a *negative caloric balance*. It is neither necessary nor desirable to create an excessively large negative caloric imbalance by exhaustive exercise or an exaggerated reduction in food intake which may produce hunger. The recommended curtailment in daily food ingestion is 500 to 1000 calories.[8,11] A daily deficit of 500 calories could lead to a potential loss of 1 pound per week (3,500 cal. = 1 lb. fat). The diet should be balanced with approximately 15 to 20% protein, no more than 30% fat, and the rest carbohydrate. It is best to spread food ingestion over the course of three or more meals a day to aid in digestion and to curtail the use of highly refined sugars.

The potential reduction in fat that can be produced cumulatively through regular exercise is summarized in Figure 2.4. Holding food intake and other variables constant, a minimal 200 calories expended through the completion

200	Calories expended/exercise bout
× 4	Exercise bouts/week
800	Potential number of calories expended/week
× 52	Weeks/year
41,600	Potential number of calories expended/year
÷3,500*	Calories/pound of fat
11.9	Pounds of fat/year

* Approximately 3,500 calories equal a pound of body weight. Weight loss is not the same as fat loss, and when body weight is decreased by 1 pound it is not necessarily a pound of fat.

FIGURE 2.4. Numerical calculations demonstrating the cumulative fat-reducing effects of exercise.

of a 20-minute light-to-moderate intensity exercise task four times a week could aid in the elimination or warding off of almost 12 pounds per year. Systematic exercise can produce a shrinkage of body fat and a growth of dense muscle and articular tissue simultaneously. This can sometimes result in the maintenance or an increase in total body weight concomitant with a reduction in body fat.

Approximate caloric costs of a variety of activities are reported in Table 2.2. Exact caloric expenditure depends on environmental conditions, degree of intensity with which the task is executed, total body weight, and other physiological and psychological variables.

The heavier the body weight, the more intense the work involved in completing a specific exercise task. Unfortunately, obese people tend to burn fewer calories than do average persons, because they move slowly and with little exuberance when engaging in exercise.

TABLE 2.2
Approximate Calorie Expenditure for Various Activities

Cal./Min. Lb. of Body Wt.	Activity	Cal./Hr. Lb. of Body Wt.
.0234	House painting	1.40
.026	Carpentry	1.56
.031	Farming, planting, hoeing, raking	1.86
.039	Gardening, weeding	2.34
.045	Pick and shovel work	2.70
.050	Chopping wood	3.00
.062	Gardening, digging	3.72
.0078	Sleeping	0.47
.0079	Resting in bed	0.47
.0080	Sitting, normally	0.48
.0080	Sitting, reading	0.48
.0089	Lying, quietly	0.54
.0093	Sitting, eating	0.56
.0096	Sitting, playing cards	0.58
.0094	Standing, normally	0.56
.011	Classwork, lecture	0.66
.012	Conversing	0.72
.012	Sitting, writing	0.72
.016	Standing, light activity	0.96
.020	Driving a car	1.20
.028	Cleaning windows	1.68
.024	Sweeping floors	1.40
.044	Walking downstairs	—
.116	Walking upstairs	—
.014	Lecturing	0.84

TABLE 2.2 (*Continued*)

Cal./Min. Lb. of Body Wt.	Activity	Cal./Hr. Lb. of Body Wt.
.023	Volleyball	1.40
.026	Playing Ping Pong	1.56
.033	Calisthenics	1.98
.033	Bicycling on level roads	1.98
.036	Golfing	2.16
.046	Playing tennis	2.76
.047	Playing basketball	2.82
.069	Playing squash	4.14
.100	Running long distance	6.00
.156	Sprinting	—
	Swimming	
.032	Breast stroke 20 yd./min.	—
.064	Breast stroke 40 yd./min.	—
.026	Back stroke 25 yd./min.	—
.056	Back stroke 40 yd./min.	—
.058	Crawl 45 yd./min.	—
.071	Crawl 55 yd./min.	—
.033	Walking on level	1.98
.093	Running on level (jogging)	5.60
.01	Fill-in constant for time unaccounted for (if not completely inactive such as sleeping or resting)	0.60

EXAMPLE: 150 pound man sitting and reading for 60 min. = 150 × .008 × 60 = 72 calories expended, or 1 hr. = 150 × .48 × 1 = 72 calories.

(From *Principles of Modern Physical Education, Health, and Recreation* by Updyke and Johnson, copyright © 1970 by Holt, Rinehart & Winston, Inc. Used with the permission of Holt, Rinehart & Winston, Inc.)

Contrary to popular opinion, appetite does not necessarily increase linearly with an increase in daily caloric expenditure (Figure 2.5). In experiments with both animals and human beings voluntary food intake was actually greater at the extremely low levels of daily caloric output than at moderately higher ones.[11] Within the range of normal energy expenditure, regulation of food intake is sensitive and precise. Intensification of daily exercise evokes increments in food intake, but not to the extent that a positive caloric imbalance results. Sedentary living seems to produce regulatory food intake disturbances that give rise to caloric intakes beyond need. At the extremely high levels of daily caloric output from exhaustive exercise (6000 calories), food intake remains somewhat below the level needed by the body to maintain its high energy expenditure.

A combination of moderate exercise and food curtailment is not an artificial or synthetic method of losing weight. The success of this type of obesity

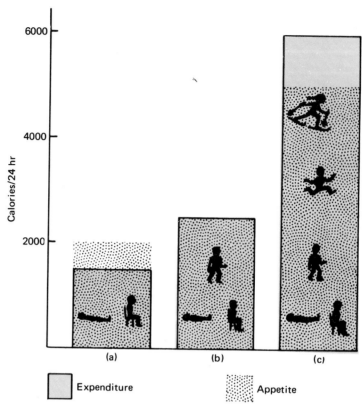

FIGURE 2.5. Appetite in relation to caloric expenditure. For most sedentary persons, caloric intake tends to exceed caloric expenditure (a). With increasing physical activity (b), a balance seems to be attained between appetite and caloric output. At extremely high levels of caloric output (c), caloric intake seems to fall below the caloric expenditure. (From *Textbook of Work Physiology* by Astrand and Rodahl, copyright 1970. Used with permission of McGraw-Hill Book Company.)

control program depends in part upon the knowledge of caloric values of varying foods and of exercises. Faithful adherence to such a program is more demanding and difficult to swallow than a reducing pill.

Rather than neglecting completely the weight problem of the excessively thin, it is recommended that ectomorphs who desire to gain weight incorporate a low caloric expenditure exercise program designed to enhance growth of muscle, bone, and joint tissue, and increase food intake.

REFERENCES

1. Adams, William C., et al. *Foundations of Physical Activity.* Champaign, Ill.: Stipes Publishing Company, 1968.
2. Astrand, O., and K. Rodahl. *Textbook of Work Physiology.* New York: McGraw-Hill Book Co., Inc., 1970.

3. Bogert, L., and G. Briggs. *Nutrition and Physical Fitness*. Philadelphia: W. B. Saunders Company, 1966.
4. Corbin, Charles B., et al. *Concepts in Physical Education: With Laboratories and Experiments*. Dubuque, Iowa: Wm. C. Brown Co., Publishers, 1970.
5. deVries, Herbert A. *Physiology of Exercise for Physical Education and Athletics*. Dubuque, Iowa: Wm. C. Brown Co., Publishers, 1966.
6. Ismail, A. H. Body Composition and Relationships to Physical Activity. In H. B. Falls (Editor), *Exercise Physiology*. New York: The Academic Press, 1968.
7. Johnson, Perry B., et al. *Physical Education: A Problem-Solving Approach to Health and Fitness*. New York: Holt, Rinehart & Winston, 1966.
8. Johnson, Perry B. Metabolism and Weight Control. *Journal of Health, Physical Education and Recreation*, 32:39–40, 1968.
9. Kraus, Hans, and Wilhelm Raab. *Hypokinetic Disease*. Springfield, Ill.: Charles C Thomas, Publisher, 1961.
10. Mayer, Jean. The Best Diet is Exercise. *The New York Times Magazine*, April 25, 1965.
11. Mayer, Jean. *Overweight*. Englewood Cliffs, N.J.: Prentice-Hall, Inc., 1968.
12. Updyke, Wynn F., and Perry Johnson. *Principles of Modern Physical Education, Health, and Recreation*. New York: Holt, Rinehart & Winston, 1970.
13. Van Huss, Wayne, et al. *Physical Activity in Modern Living*. Englewood Cliffs, N.J.: Prentice-Hall, Inc., 1960.

CHAPTER THREE

The O₂ Transport System

*In strenuous exercise, the demands for oxygen are greatly increased,
and the tireless (heart) pump responds accordingly. The heart of a
trained athlete in action may pump over 30 quarts of blood per minute—enough blood to carry fifteen times as much oxygen from his
lungs. This superior oxygen-capturing power distinguishes the
trained man.*

ARTHUR STEINHAUS

BLOOD AND CIRCULATION

The O_2 transport system includes the blood, blood vessels, heart, and
lungs. Blood is seldom thought of as a body organ because of its mobility.
It consists of liquid plasma, solids in the form of blood cells and proteins, and
gases such as carbon dioxide (CO_2) and oxygen (O_2). It is transported to all
body parts through an extensive network of blood vessels referred to as the
arterial system. Following entry into tissue capillaries, blood is returned to
the heart by means of the *venous system*, which is composed of small veins that
flow into larger veins eventually emptying into the heart. It has been estimated that the blood travels through the body's 60,000 miles of blood vessels
about 1500 times a day.

Blood moves readily from a high to a low pressure area. Venous return is
inherently handicapped, because blood pressure is lower in veins than
arteries. Approximately 50% of the total blood volume is in the veins during
rest.[2] Owing to the force of gravity, pressure bears down on venous blood
(*hydrostatic pressure*) resulting in a tendency for the blood to pool in the extremities and mid-section. Repetitive muscle contraction squeezes blood
from the capillaries into veins, reducing hydrostatic pressure. This muscle
pumping, termed *peripheral heart action*, enhances the blood flow to the heart.
Small valves located on the lining of the veins help prevent any backward
precipitation of blood.

27

Another natural aid to venous return is the *abdominothoracic pump*. The descent of the diaphragm during inspiration intensifies pressure in the abdomen and simultaneously diminishes thoracic pressure. The resulting pressure gradient (higher pressure in the mid-section than the chest) speeds the passage of blood through this area.[8]

THE HEART

The heart is a maintainer of human life. It is a uniquely constructed and powerful muscle with two sides or loops, each acting as a separate pump (Figure 3.1). Both sides have blood reception and ejection chambers. The thin-walled receiving chamber, called the *atrium*, has little contractile power, because its primary function is merely the transfer of blood to the *ventricle*. The ventricle is the larger and more thickly lined chamber that must contract forcefully to discharge blood from itself.

The heart beats or contracts in a rhythmical manner. Cellular fibers of the *myocardium*, the heart tissue, are connected in series. When one fiber is excited the action potential or stimulation spreads to the other cells causing a single contraction. When the walls contract, a rising pressure within the chambers forces the blood through one-way valves into established arterial pathways. Following ejection, pressure is reduced and blood enters the heart.

Heart muscle is at rest when the ventricles are filling with blood, called *diastole*. *Systole* is the period during which the myocardium is at work pumping blood. The left ventricle must eject blood with sufficient power to enable it to travel freely through the aorta. Its pressure and forcefulness of contraction must be more intense than those of the right ventricle which drives the blood into the lungs.

The volume of blood the heart supplies to itself depends on myocardial demands. Coronary blood flow can be increased five times the resting level during periods of cardiac stress. The magnified blood supply and the myocardium's high degree of O_2 extraction from the blood (70 to 80%) ensure adequate provision for the heart's metabolic requirements during strenuous muscular work.[2]

CARDIOVASCULAR EFFICIENCY

The effectiveness of the coronary arteries and other blood vessels in transferring blood is highly dependent on their resiliency and *lumen* or diameter. When the diameter of a blood vessel is decreased because of degeneration or fatty deposits, the movement of blood is hampered. The pressure needed to maintain a given rate of blood flow from the heart must be increased.[11]

The heart will pump only the blood present in it. The *cardiac output* (Q) is the volume of blood ejected from the heart in one minute. It is a composite of *stroke volume* or amount of blood discharged with one contraction, and heart rate or the number of contractions per minute. When the venous system is efficient and the left ventricle dilates readily to receive oxygenated

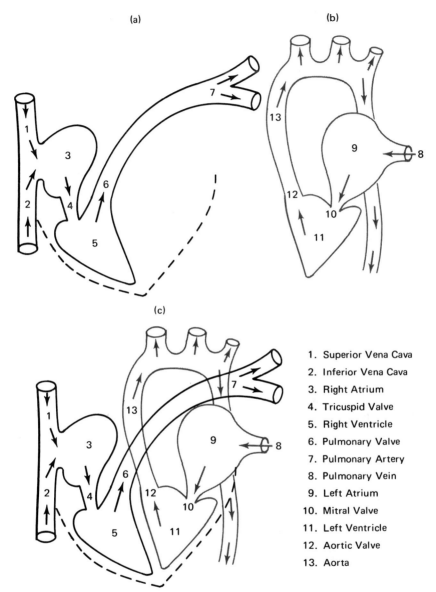

FIGURE 3.1. Heart structure and cardiac cycle. (a) Left side of the heart; (b) right side of the heart; (c) whole heart. Blood flows into the right atrium from the superior and inferior vena cava, the two largest veins of the body. It passes through the tricuspid valve into the right ventricle, which drives it through the pulmonary arteries into the lungs. Following pulmonary processing, oxygenated blood flows through the pulmonary veins into the atrium on the left side of the heart. The left ventricle distends as it receives blood traveling through the mitral valve, located between the ventricle and the atrium. The propulsion of the blood from the left ventricle into the aorta, the body's main artery, is the final phase of the cardiac cycle.

TABLE 3.1
Cardiac Output, Stroke Volume, and Heart Rate (Upright Position)
for an Untrained and a Trained Person

	Cardiac Output (l.)		Stroke Volume (ml.)		Heart Rate (beats/min.)	
	Resting	Maximal	Resting	Maximal	Resting	Maximal
Untrained person	5.1	18.5	60	100	85	198
Trained person	6.4	28.0	100	150	64	185

TABLE 3.2
Effects of Stroke Volume and Heart Rate on Cardiac Output

Subject	Stroke Volume (l.)	× Heart Rate (beats/min.) =		Cardiac Output (l.)
A	0.17	120	=	20
B	0.13	160	=	20

blood from the lungs a relatively long diastole (and thus large ventricular blood volume) can be expected. Stroke volume is magnified provided the myocardium contracts forcefully to propel all the blood from the ventricles. If the pressure in the aorta and branching arteries is greater than that within the left ventricle, blood flow is resisted[8] (Table 3.1).

When cardiovascular mechanisms influencing stroke volume operate effectively, heart rate is low. Highly conditioned individuals have attained resting heart rates of 40 beats per minute. If these mechanisms are inefficient the heart compensates for the resulting reduction in stroke volume by beating faster (Table 3.2). Despite the same 20-liter cardiac output, subject A, who has the greater stroke volume, is operating with a greater blood reserve and less cardiac stress (40 fewer beats/minute) than is B.

When the heart rate approaches 180 beats per minute during strenuous muscle activity, stroke volume becomes so drastically reduced (owing to the shortness of diastole) that subsequent increases in heart rate can no longer compensate for blood losses. Thus, the most that cardiac output can be heightened through an increase in heart rate alone is two to two and one-half times the resting level.[8]

RESPIRATORY FUNCTIONING

Respiration is simply the exchange of oxygen for carbon dioxide within the body. *External respiration*, which occurs in the lungs (Figure 3.2), depends on the amount of air inspired per minute (*pulmonary ventilation*) and the diffusion capacity of the lungs. Oxygen composes approximately 15% of the

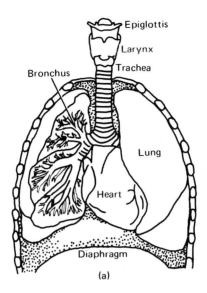

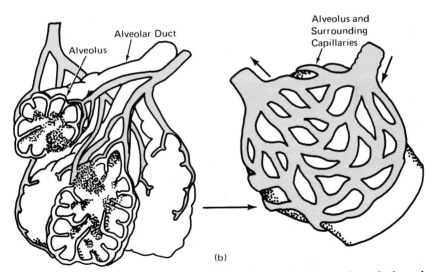

FIGURE 3.2. Pulmonary circuit. (a) Blood enters both lungs through the pulmonary arteries which branch into capillaries. Minute alveoli, the thin-walled air sacs which branch from larger air-carrying tubes entering the lungs, contact the capillaries. Here O_2 exchanges for CO_2, which is then expired. (b) An alveolus: there are approximately 300 million alveoli within the lungs, each of which is covered with a network of capillaries. The capillary system of the lungs is the richest of all the body organs.

TABLE 3.3

Pulmonary Measures at Rest and During Strenuous Muscle Work

	Tidal Volume (l. air)	Breathing Rate (breaths/min.)	Pulmonary Ventilation (l. air/min.)
Rest	0.5	12	6
Strenuous muscular work	1.4–3.6	50	70–180

air we breathe. Thus, the volume of air inhaled per breath (*tidal volume*) and the number of breaths per minute are the major pulmonary determinants of oxygen consumption (Table 3.3).

Air intake and the diffusion of gases within the lungs are proportional to the size of the lungs, the thickness of the pulmonary membranes, the force of the respiratory muscles (diaphragm, intercostals, and abdominals), and the compliance or elasticity of the chest wall.[3] Naturally, lung disease and foreign substances that enter the lungs, such as cigarette smoke, oppose air flow and reduce respiratory functioning.

During rest the volumes of air and blood within the lungs are minimal. The carbon dioxide-oxygen exchange does not take place at all pulmonary levels. Both tidal volume and cardiac output are increased significantly when working muscles demand more O_2. More lung tissue is activated to handle the larger air and blood volumes. *Vascularization*, an increase in the number of functioning capillary beds, within the lungs magnifies the carbon dioxide taken from the blood and the oxygen processed into it; more so than any increase in the speed of the gas exchange among alveoli and lung capillaries.[10] After oxygen consumption reaches a level that is 40% of the maximal aerobic capacity during muscular activity, increases in pulmonary gas diffusion are minimal.

INTERNAL RESPIRATION

Internal respiration is the gas exchange among body cells and local capillaries (Figure 3.3). The number of functioning capillary beds within a muscle is proportional to its degree of metabolism. One twentieth to one fiftieth of a muscle's total capillary vessels are open during rest.[2] Vascularization during physical activity can heighten the volume of blood passing through muscles to 15 times the resting level. Blood remains within capillaries for a period of one to two seconds regardless of degree of muscle activation.[2] The increased capillary surface area facilitates the transference of metabolic material across capillary and cellular membranes by shortening the distance these nutrients must travel to be diffused. Thus, the oxygen extracted from the blood by muscle tissue can become as high as 80%. Greater concentrations of carbon dioxide in muscle cells and a rise in arterial blood pressure

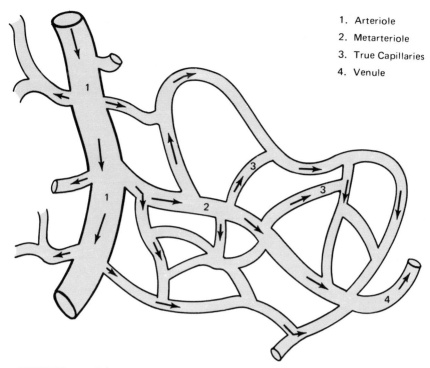

1. Arteriole
2. Metarteriole
3. True Capillaries
4. Venule

FIGURE 3.3. Muscle capillary unit. True capillaries are only 1 mm. in length and 0.4 mm. in width. Sometimes they are so narrow that red blood cells must change shape to squeeze through them.

also aid internal respiration.[9] The oxygen content of venous blood in active muscle is approximately four times less than when the same tissues are inactive. Results of studies indicate that the improved cardiac output and blood flow through muscle are the crucial factors in the adjustment to moderate and heavy work.[8]

A constriction in the blood vessels of body organs (liver, kidneys, spleen, intestines, and stomach) during exercise reduces their blood supply (Figure 3.4). Thus more blood becomes available to working muscles as well as skin. The need to conduct the heat produced during sustained muscular activity from inside to the surface of the body for exchange with the environment causes the intensification of blood flow in skin.

OXYGEN CONSUMPTION, CARDIAC COST, AND RECOVERY ABILITY

O$_2$ transport mechanisms are in operation during rest because the body consumes approximately 0.25 liter of oxygen per minute. Greater demands are made on the heart, lungs, blood, and blood vessels during periods of stress, and Vo$_2$ increases somewhat linearly with oxygen requirements. In

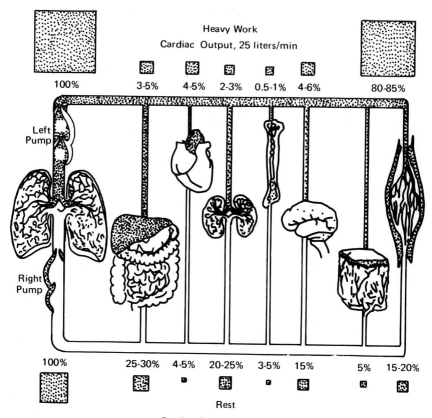

FIGURE 3.4. Blood flow during rest and heavy exercise. Cardiac output may be increased fivefold when changing from rest to strenuous exercise. The above figures indicate the relative distribution of the blood to the various organs at rest (lower scale) and during exercise (upper scale). During exercise the circulating blood is primarily directed to the muscles. These percentages are based on the minute volume of blood flow. (From *Textbook of Work Physiology* by Astrand and Rodahl, copyright 1970. Used with permission of McGraw-Hill Book Company.)

attempting to meet work demands, a person with an ineffective O_2 transport system may consume as little as 1 liter of oxygen per minute (as compared to an average Vo_2 range of 2.5 to 3.0). Certain trained men have developed the capacity to consume 6 liters of oxygen per minute. In performing strenuous muscular work in a steady state, the rate of breathing seldom reaches maximal levels. This seems to indicate that a subaverage Vo_2 is probably due to the rate at which oxygenated blood can be pumped from the heart (cardiac output) rather than to the failure of external (or internal) respiratory variables.[10,11]

Response of heart rate to muscular work demands is a practical and objective indicator of the efficiency of the O_2 transport system. Resting heart rate provides a measure of how the heart must work to maintain homeostasis. A heart pump that has a resting rate of 60 beats per minute has the potential to contract 38,000 fewer times a day than one with a rate of 80. Heart rate measured while performing at a steady state is, with certain exceptions, directly proportional to cardiac output and oxygen consumption.[2,8] The increase in heart rate from resting level is termed *cardiac cost*. *Recovery ability* is the time required for the heart rate to return to resting level following the cessation of work stress. The lower the cost and the quicker the recovery, the more efficient the O₂ transport system is in acquiring and transporting oxygen (and removing CO_2) for active tissue consumption during and following physical activity.

REFERENCES

1. Adams, William C., et al. *Foundations of Physical Activity*. Champaign, Ill.: Stipes Publishing Company, 1968.
2. Andersen, K. L. The Cardiovascular System in Exercise. In H. B. Falls (Editor), *Exercise Physiology*. New York: The Academic Press, 1968.
3. Astrand, O., and K. Rodahl. *Textbook of Work Physiology*. New York: McGraw-Hill Book Company, 1970.
4. Basmajian, John V. *Primary Anatomy*. Baltimore: Williams & Wilkins Co., 1970.
5. Brouha, L., and E. P. Radford. The Cardiovascular System in Muscular Activity. In W. Johnson (Editor), *Science and Medicine in Exercise and Sport*. New York: Harper & Row, Publishers, 1960.
6. Brouha, L. A. Effect of Work on the Heart. In F. F. Rosenbaum and E. L. Belknap (Editors), *Work and the Heart*. New York: Paul B. Hoeber, Inc., 1969.
7. Corbin, Charles B., et al. *Concepts in Physical Education: With Laboratories and Experiments*. Dubuque, Iowa: Wm. C. Brown Co., Publishers, 1970.
8. deVries, Herbert A. *Physiology of Exercise for Physical Education and Athletics*. Dubuque, Iowa: Wm. C. Brown Co., Publishers, 1966.
9. Johnson, Perry B., et al. *Physical Education: A Problem-Solving Approach to Health and Fitness*. New York: Holt, Rinehart & Winston, 1966.
10. Margaria, R., and P. Cartelli. The Respiratory System and Exercise. In H. B. Falls (Editor), *Exercise Physiology*. New York: The Academic Press, 1968.
11. Ricci, Benjamin. *Physical and Physiological Conditioning for Men*. Dubuque, Iowa: Wm. C. Brown Co., Publishers, 1966.
12. Ricci, Benjamin. *Physiological Basis of Human Performance*. Philadelphia: Lea & Febiger, 1967.
13. Riley, Richard L. Pulmonary Function in Relation to Exercise. In W. Johnson (Editor), *Science and Medicine in Exercise and Sports*. New York: Harper & Row, Publishers, 1960.

CHAPTER FOUR

Neuromuscular Functioning

*. . . What a disgrace it is for a man to grow old without ever seeing
the beauty and strength of which his body is capable.*

SOCRATES

The speed and beauty of movement as well as the capacity to sustain exercise
without injury depend on integrated muscle, nerve, and skeletal action.
The human skeleton protects body organs, stores calcium, and produces
red and white blood cells. It also provides a network of levers that enables
man to support, transport, and control his body, as well as to manipulate
many objects in his environment. Bone is set in motion when acted upon by
one or more muscles. However, the tension within the muscle that pulls
the bone is produced by nervous stimulation.

NERVOUS STIMULATION

The human nervous system includes the brain and spinal cord (*central
nervous system*) and the peripheral nerves that connect body parts to them.
In terms of function, the *autonomic division* of the nervous system tends to
control organic responses that are automatic, such as those involving the
functioning of the heart, kidney, liver, and blood vessels. The operation of
such organs is naturally balanced by the antagonism of autonomic nerve
inhibitors and stimulators. Activities over which man has conscious control, such as movement, speech, and thought, are regulated by the *somatic
division* of the nervous system.

A nerve is composed of one or more *neurons* or nerve cells. The primary
function of the neuron is to receive a stimulus or message and pass it to
another neuron, muscle cell, or other body cell. The nerve impulse is a
series of electrochemical changes along the cell membrane and is transferred
to other cells resulting in some type of biochemical reaction. The firing of
an impulse by a neuron is similar to a fuse carrying a spark at high speed.

Three types of neurons are involved in muscular work. The nerve cell

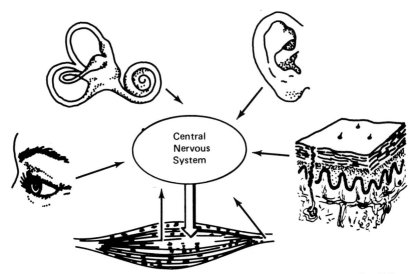

FIGURE 4.1.   The central nervous system receives information via different nerves from the various receptors.   (From *Textbook of Work Physiology* by Astrand and Rodahl, copyright 1970.   Used with permission of McGraw-Hill Book Company.)

that carries messages to the central nervous system from receptors in the joint capsules, ligaments, muscles, sense organs, viscera, and blood vessels is a *sensory* or *afferent* neuron (Figure 4.1).

The *motor* or *efferent* neuron conducts stimulation to the muscle tissue to activate it.   The transfer of nerve impulses within the brain and spinal cord is the function of *interneurons*, which connect with motor and sensory neurons as well as other interneurons.   An interneuron will provide for either *facilitation*, an acceleration in the transfer of impulses among neurons, or *inhibition*, the blocking of an impulse to be relayed to another nerve cell. Actually, perception in space and smooth performance of movement require a high degree of coordination among sensory receptors carrying impulses to the central nervous system, interneurons that are constantly exposed to facilitation and inhibition from various levels in the central nervous system, and motor neurons that stimulate muscles.

MUSCLE STRUCTURE AND ACTIVATION

Three kinds of muscle tissue exist within the body: *smooth muscle*, located within walls of various body organs; *cardiac* or heart muscle tissue; and *striated* tissue of the skeletal muscles which fasten to bones.   Tough, resilient connective tissue surrounds skeletal muscle and forms *tendon* as it branches off at its end points to insert onto another bone.   The *joint* where two or more bones articulate is the actual site of limb movement.   In the production of movement, mechanical muscle tension is transmitted through the tendon to the attaching bone (Figure 4.2).

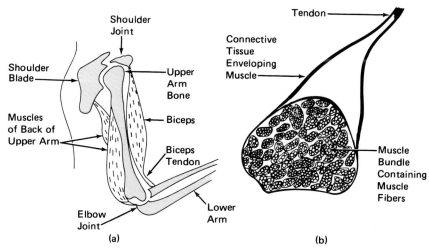

FIGURE 4.2. (a) Schematic representation of the cigar-shaped biceps inserting the lower arm at the elbow joint. (b) Cross section of biceps muscle.

The muscles of the body have Latin names (Figures 4.7 and 4.8) and vary in shape from those arranged in thin sheets (abdominals) to cigar-shaped types such as the biceps of the upper arm (Figure 4.2). The stapedius of the inner ear, only a few millimeters in length, is the smallest body muscle; the longest is usually the sartorius which extends approximately 2 feet down the thigh connecting the hip with the lower leg.

A muscle is composed of bundles of cylindrical cells in fiber form. Thousands of these fibers, ranging in diameter from microscopic to those as large as a human hair, are arranged within each bundle. Some are quite long and may run the entire length of the muscle. The individual cells, muscle bundles, and the whole muscle are covered with connective tissue.

Each fiber has a membrane containing intracellular fluid. This fluid contains myoglobin, glycogen, and fat (foods utilized in cellular activity), phosphates which are crucial energy liberators, and *myofibrils* which are small rodlike structures. The precise nature by which a muscle contracts or shortens is still not completely understood. However, it is believed that bands of protein rods (*actin* and *myosin*) arranged lengthwise and in parallel in the myofibrils, under proper signal from the motor neuron and in the presence of energy producers, slide together causing the muscle fiber to shorten for a brief instant. When enough fibers shorten simultaneously, the muscle contracts.

Motor neurons entering the muscle bundle separate into many twiglike branches, each stimulating a muscle cell. A group of muscle fibers connected to the branches of a motor neuron is called a *motor unit* (Figure 4.3). The number of fibers within a motor unit varies from five to 2000.[3] The fibers of a motor unit are scattered and intermingled with those of other units.

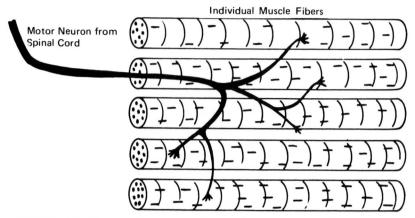

FIGURE 4.3. Schematic representation of the motor unit. The motor neuron enters the muscle from the central nervous system and branches into many subconnections, each of which innervates a single muscle fiber.

When stimulation reaches *threshold* level, that is, the intensity necessary to warrant responses, all muscle fibers of the motor unit contract. If the stimulation is not adequate none of the muscle fibers of the unit will contract. At no time is there a partial firing in which only a portion of the unit's muscle fibers act. This firing or non-firing is termed the *all or none law*.

MUSCLE STRENGTH AND ENDURANCE

The force of a muscle contraction depends on the number of motor units in operation and their frequency of firing.[2] When a single low intensity stimulus allows a single firing of a minimal number of motor units the muscle will merely twitch due to the shortening of a small number of muscle fibers. With a greater degree and rate of stimulation more units come into and remain in action. A limb moves because an adequate number of motor units fire at a sufficient frequency to cause the shortening of enough fibers to pull the bone to which the muscle inserts. If the limb is to move against a resistance, the muscle must render a contraction of higher magnitude. The same motor units are engaged with greater frequency and, in addition, higher threshold units are recruited to allow more muscle fibers to contract simultaneously, thus producing more muscle tension.

Muscle *strength* is simply the maximum tension a muscle can exert under a set of prescribed circumstances. It is highly dependent on the composition of muscle tissue and the number of muscle cells that may be willfully innervated.

A small number of motor units firing at a low frequency seems to be a significant factor in the limited strength of a muscle. Muscle training is believed to reduce inhibition and to increase facilitation in motor units. This results in the mobilization of higher threshold motor neurons as well as an acceleration in motor unit firing, causing the muscle fibers to contract with greater synchronization. The influence of the nervous system in triggering muscle response may help explain why strength levels in some individuals vary from test to test, and why the cross-sectional area of the muscle is not a perfectly valid predictor of its strength.[3]

Isotonic or *dynamic* strength involves tension required to move a resistance through full (or close to full) range of joint motion. An isotonic contraction is one in which the muscle shortens despite the fact that the level of muscle tension, which depends on the magnitude of the resistance, remains constant. Dynamic strength is most commonly measured by the amount of weight resistance the limb is capable of moving.

Isometric or *static* strength is the maximum tension a muscle can produce at a determined angle of joint motion. The muscle fibers shorten to a spe-

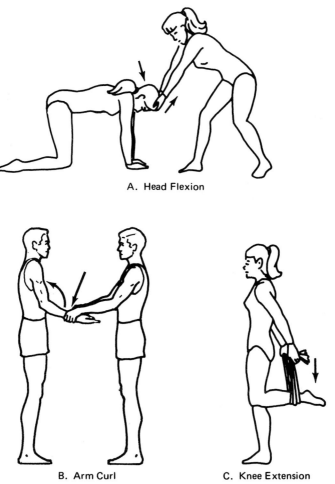

A. Head Flexion

B. Arm Curl   C. Knee Extension

FIGURE 4.4. Examples of isometric exercises.

cific point, while continuing to build a maximal or nearly maximal tension level during an isometric contraction. Power, sometimes confused with strength, is the degree of explosiveness or speed with which a muscle can contract (Figure 4.4).

Endurance, the ability of a muscle or a muscle group to persist in contraction, is also classified as dynamic (capacity to continue isotonic contractions) and static (capacity to sustain isometric activity). Dynamic endurance is frequently measured by the number of times a limb can perform a movement against a specific resistance, whereas static endurance is determined by the length of time a limb can hold a particular position.

When a muscle has strength enough to contract against a resistance by utilizing a small number of motor units it allows the unused motor units to rest. This group may take over later allowing the first group of units to recover. By rotating in this manner, waste buildup is gradual, and the movement can be continued for a much longer period of time. Thus, strong muscles usually have higher endurance levels than do weak ones.[13]

Because oxygen and fuel requirements diminish when fewer motor units (and thus fewer muscle fibers) operate, the blood supply to sedentary muscle tissue is reduced. When muscle fibers are brought into action systematically for longer periods of time through training, muscle vascularization occurs, resulting in an increase in the volume of blood supplied to the muscle. The oxygen consumption capacity of the working muscle improves and the muscle grows in aerobic and anaerobic capacities. Local vascularization appears to be the primary factor in muscle endurance, but the volume of oxygenated blood available to working muscle tissues depends on other oxygen transport mechanisms (see Chapter Three).

It has been theorized that activation of capillaries and growth of connective tissue within a muscle cause *hypertrophy*, increase in muscle size. *Atrophy* or muscle shrinkage results from a reduction in blood supply and connective tissue. Declines in endurance, strength, and power are characteristic of muscle atrophy.

CONCENTRIC AND ECCENTRIC MOVEMENT

Muscle tension is exerted through concentric or eccentric movements. A *concentric* movement occurs when the muscle shortens to move against resistance as when a limb moves against gravity. The lengthening of muscle and the return of the limb to its original position can take place by two methods. One is to relax the muscle and allow gravitational pull rather than muscle action to move the limb. The second is *eccentric* movement, that is, to lengthen the muscle gradually from its shortened state and thus control the movement pattern. In chinning, concentric movement occurs when the biceps (anterior upper arm muscle) contracts causing flexion of the elbows and the pulling of the chin over the cross-bar. The lowering of the body to the extended elbow hanging position could occur by relaxing the biceps and dropping with gravity, or eccentrically by gradually lengthening the biceps muscle. Eccentric movement involves utilization of muscle tissues. Thus, muscle training should include eccentric as well as concentric movement to attain maximum neuromuscular benefits.

JOINT AND MUSCLE ACTION

The physiology of the articular system (joints) ensures safe and efficient movement. *Joint ligaments* are the bands of connective tissue that hold the bones together with security, but allow *flexibility*, the capacity of the joint to attain full range of motion. *Synovial fluid* lubricates the joint. *Cartilage*, a connective tissue covering the articular surfaces of bones, seems to aid joints to absorb shocks. It is crucial that cartilage, tendons, and ligaments within major body joints remain strong and resilient so as to support and move body parts effectively and with less chance of strain and disability.

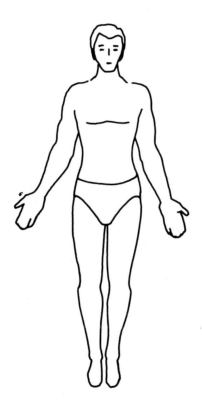

FIGURE 4.5. Anatomical standing position.

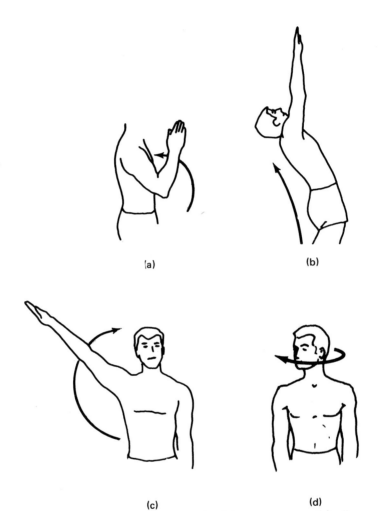

(a)   (b)

(c)   (d)

FIGURE 4.6. Examples of major joint movements: (a) elbow flexion; (b) back hyperextension; (c) shoulder abduction; (d) neck rotation.

Knowledge of joint and muscle action should better enable one to scrutinize human movements, and thus to select exercises that foster joint strength and flexibility and muscle strength and endurance.

Joint movement can be described in terms of the *anatomical standing position*; an erect standing position, face forward, arms and legs extended with the palms of the hands turned forward (Figure 4.5). *Flexion* is the movement of a body segment directly forward or backward so that either its front or back surface approaches the front or back surface of an adjacent body segment. Joint *extension* involves returning from flexion to the anatomical position. The continuation of extension beyond the anatomical position is termed *hyperextension*. The moving of a limb laterally from the body is *abduction* and the reverse is *adduction*, that is, moving from abduction to the anatomical position. *Rotation* is the turning of a bone inward or outward on its axis (Figure 4.6).

An *agonist* or primary mover is a muscle responsible for providing the tension that results in a basic joint movement such as flexion. Figures 4.7 and 4.8 give the location of the major agonists and the major joint actions they produce. *Synergists* are muscles that aid primary movers in the production of a specific joint movement. Gross body movements usually involve the activation of several synergists. A muscle or muscle group that anchors a body area so that a mover has a firm base of support upon which to pull is called a *stabilizer*. Because muscle tension tends to pull both ends of the muscle toward the center, stabilizers contract to counteract the pull at the opposite end of the bone from where the tension causes joint movement. When the biceps contracts, stabilizers in the shoulder tend to hold the upper arm bone firmly in the shoulder joint as the elbow flexes.

An *antagonist* muscle causes movement opposite that caused by the agonist. Flexors and extensors, and abductors and adductors are antagonistic muscle groups. Because an agonist tends to pull in one direction, antagonistic muscle pairs are often arranged on opposite sides of a bone so that the joint can bend back and forth.[13] Relaxation in the antagonist accompanies the contraction of an agonist. Most people cannot distinguish whether a joint movement involves an eccentric contraction of an agonist or a concentric contraction of an antagonist. The following example should help resolve this confusion. In performing a push-up the elbow flexor (biceps) hardly comes into action despite a flexing movement in the elbow when the body is lowered to the ground prior to pushing up. Actually, gravity is working to pull the body down rather than the tension within the biceps. The push-up agonist (triceps), which extends the elbow, contracts eccentrically to brake and control the downward movement of the body.

In the successful performance of even the elementary joint movements, several muscles support and assist the primary mover. The amount and timing of tension in these different muscles as well as the inhibition of antagonists result from a complex integration of responses within the nervous system.

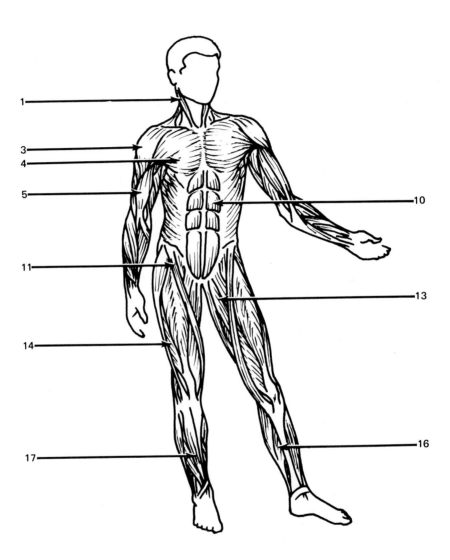

MUSCLE	PRIMARY JOINT ACTION

1. Sternomastoid — Head support, flexion & rotation

3. Deltoid (3 heads) — Arm flexion; extension hyperextension; inward & outward rotation.

4. Pectoralis Major — Arm flexion & inward arm rotation.

5. Biceps — Elbow flexion.

10. Abdominals
    Rectus Abdominis — Support upper abdomen & lower ribs;
    Transversalis — rotation of rib cage; spine & upper
    Internal Oblique — trunk flexion
    External Oblique

11. Hip Flexors
    Illiopsoas — Hip flexion & knee flexion.
    Pectineus
    Sartorius

13. Hip Adductors
    Adductor Longus — Hip adduction.
    Gracilis
    Adductor Brevis
    Adductor Magnus

14. Quadriceps
    Rectus Femoris — Hip flexion & knee extension
    Vastus Medialis
    Vastus Lateralis
    Vastus Intermedius

16. Ankle Extensors
    Gastrocnemius — Ankle extension (plantar flexion)
    Soleus

17. Ankle Flexors
    Extensor Hallucis — Ankle flexion (dorsal flexion)
    Longus
    Anterior Tibial

FIGURE 4.7. Major muscles and primary joint actions: anterior view.

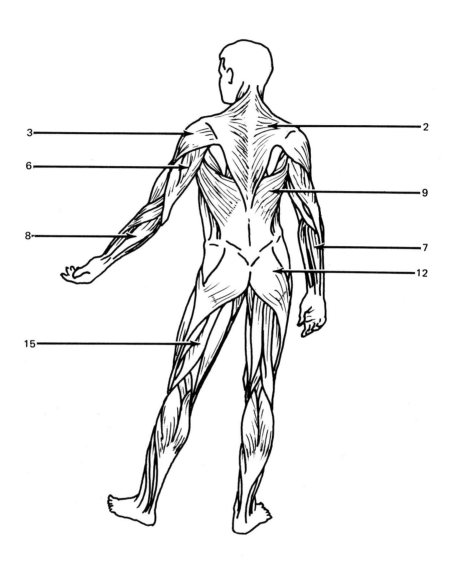

MUSCLE	PRIMARY JOINT ACTION
2. Trapezius	Head extension and rotation.
3. Deltoid (3 heads)	Arm flexion; extension hyper-extension; inward & outward rotation.
6. Triceps	Elbow extension.
7. Wrist Flexors	Wrist flexion.
8. Wrist Extensors	Wrist extension.
9. Latissimus Dorsi (lats)	Arm adduction & extension.
12. Gluteals Gluteus Maximus Gluteus Medius Gluteus Minimus	Hip extension & abduction.
15. Hamstrings Semitendinosus Semimembranosus Biceps Femoris	Hip extension & knee flexion.

FIGURE 4.8. Major muscles and primary joint actions: posterior view.

REFERENCES

1. Adams, William C., et al. *Foundations of Physical Activity.* Champaign, Ill.: Stipes Publishing Company, 1968.
2. Amussen, E. The Neuromuscular System and Exercise. In H. B. Falls (Editor), *Exercise Physiology.* New York: The Academic Press, 1968.
3. Astrand, O., and K. Rodahl. *Textbook of Work Physiology.* New York: McGraw-Hill Book Co., 1970.
4. Basmajian, John V. *Primary Anatomy.* Baltimore: Williams & Wilkins Company, 1970.
5. Broer, M. R. *Efficiency of Human Movement.* Philadelphia: W. B. Saunders Co., 1960.
6. Corbin, Charles B., et al. *Concepts in Physical Education: With Laboratories and Experiments.* Dubuque, Iowa: Wm. C. Brown Co., Publishers, 1970.
7. deVries, Herbert A. *Physiology of Exercise for Physical Education and Athletics.* Dubuque, Iowa: Wm. C. Brown Co., Publishers, 1966.
8. Johnson, Perry B., et al. *Physical Education: A Problem-Solving Approach to Health and Fitness.* New York: Holt, Rinehart, & Winston, 1966.
9. Loofbourrow, G. N. Neuromuscular Integration. In W. Johnson (Editor), *Science and Medicine of Exercise and Sports.* New York: Harper & Row, Publishers, 1960.
10. Mathews, D., and E. Fox. *The Physiological Basis of Physical Education and Athletics.* Philadelphia: W. B. Saunders Co., 1971.
11. MacConaill, M., and J. V. Basmajian. *Muscles and Movements: A Basis for Human Kinesiology.* Baltimore: William & Wilkins Company, 1969.
12. Ricci, Benjamin. *Physiological Basis of Human Performance.* Philadelphia: Lea & Febiger, 1967.
13. Sorani, Robert. *Circuit Training.* Dubuque, Iowa: Wm. C. Brown Co., Publishers, 1966.
14. Taylor, H. L. Exercise and Metabolism. In W. Johnson (Editor), *Science and Medicine of Exercise and Sports.* New York: Harper & Row, Publishers, 1960.
15. Tuttle, W., and Byron Schotteluis. *Textbook of Physiology.* St. Louis: The C. V. Mosby Company, 1961.
16. Updyke, Wynn F., and Perry Johnson. *Principles of Modern Physical Education, Health, and Recreation.* New York: Holt, Rinehart, & Winston, 1970.
17. Wells, K. F. *Kinesiology.* Philadelphia: W. B. Saunders Co., 1966.

CHAPTER FIVE

Toward the Development
and Maintenance of
Optimal Physical Fitness

That which is used develops, and that which is not used wastes away.
HIPPOCRATES

Exercise is simply the performance of muscular work. In physiological terms it is any muscle activity that increases heart, lung, blood, blood vessel, and muscle metabolism. Most of man's exercise in the past involved occupational and household tasks. Due to the devices of the machine age the total energy expenditure from required work duties is quite low for the majority of the population in the United States. Atrophy and weakening of muscles, loss of joint strength and flexibility, reduction of blood circulation in the lungs and muscles, weakening of the heart pump, body fat increment, and a reduction in muscular work capacity are physiological adaptations to prolonged inactivity.[1] Fortunately, they are not permanent, and, if he desires, man can enhance his physical fitness level through regular exercise within bounds set by heredity.

Implementation of the following principles, precautions, and recommendations will assure safe and effective exercise-fitness programs for men and women of varying ages and fitness levels.

PRINCIPLES OF EXERCISE FOR OPTIMAL PHYSICAL FITNESS

Readiness. All individuals who exercise should be in a state of physiological and psychological readiness. A thorough medical examination is recommended prior to commencing a regular exercise program, especially for an older or more sedentary person. If possible it should be supplemented with fitness evaluations which provide feedback pertaining to physiological needs (see Laboratory Workbook). These appraisals will also aid in deciding a beginning exercise intensity level and provide a baseline for objectively measuring the results of regular activity.

Specificity. Physiological changes produced through exercise are specific to the intensity, duration, and types of activities performed. Generally speaking, short bursts of highly demanding muscular work seem to develop muscle-joint strength and endurance best. Aerobic power (Vo_2) is best developed through exercises that tax large muscle masses fully for 3- to 5-minute periods, whereas the improvement of the O_2 transport system's capacity to handle prolonged muscular work utilizing the largest percentage of maximal Vo_2 would require sustained exercise for as long as 30 minutes.[2]

Balance. No exercise regimen can be universally prescribed for all persons. An athlete training for competition is sometimes required to exercise strenuously more than once a day, whereas another person may engage in moderate exercise such as jogging several times a week. Fitness goals should be realistic and in line with one's physiological nature. Frustration, unhappiness, and even disability could result from an exercise program that is beyond a person's capacities.

A specialized program, such as exercise of an atrophied muscle, may be warranted when weaknesses exist. However, if a major fitness deficiency does not exist, a balanced program should be designed to enhance total fitness. A well-rounded basic program for all regardless of age or sex would include exercises designed to develop the O_2 transport system and major muscle-joint areas of the body (back, mid-section, chest, arms, and legs). In cases of uncertainty about fitness evaluation or program design, a qualified physical education specialist should be consulted for guidance and direction.

Overload. In a controlled laboratory experiment, systematic performance of a set exercise task caused a gradual reduction in the cardiac cost of the activity of about 20 heart beats per minute. Subsequent performances of this exercise task failed to yield further reductions in cardiac cost. However, after the subject engaged regularly in a more stressful exercise bout, the original task was again performed with a drop in cardiac cost well below 20 heart beats.[2] Thus, an intensification of exercise demands produced adaptations in the O_2 transport system that were reflected in the gradual decrements in cardiac cost. The consistent upgrading in the metabolic requirements of exercise is commonly called *overload*. Progressive overload results in an improved exercise performance potential. Figure 5.1 depicts the effect of overload on muscular work capacity.

Overload to O_2 transport mechanisms is provided by any exercise that produces a *critical threshold*, that is, a heart rate at which improvements in cardiovascular-respiratory mechanisms occur and below which adaptations fail to occur.

Muscle and joint overload can be applied by systematically increasing the (1) speed of muscle contractions, (2) resistance against which the limb must

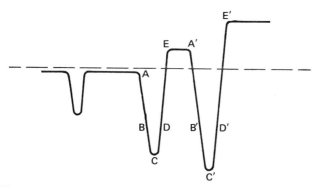

FIGURE 5.1. Muscular work curve. The letters represent the various parts of the curve: A, the potential for muscular work; B, muscular work performance; C, cessation of work; D, recovery from muscular work; and E, *exaltation* or the new capacity for muscular work following adaptation by body fitness mechanisms to previous work demands. As an individual consistently increases B (overload), E will continually rise to a higher-than-previous level. Exaltation depends on the degree of overload resulting from intensity and/or duration of work. Work intensity is the more significant overload variable in that it can create great stress to fitness mechanisms in a short time period. (From Problems of the Fight for Longevity, by D. Mateeff. *Quest*, III, 41–50, 1964.)

move, (3) number of movements against a set resistance, and (4) length of time a muscle is held in contraction.

It should be realized that the relationship between overload and its effects is not completely linear. Doubling exercise intensity or duration does not necessarily double fitness benefits. For example, if two hours of exercise per week produces V_{O_2} gains of 0.4 l. oxygen/min., four hours of the same activity will not result in a V_{O_2} increase of 0.8 l. oxygen/min.

The rate and magnitude of physiological change resulting from exercise vary among individuals. The more the functioning state of fitness mechanisms is reduced below optimal level, the greater the potential for improvement. Obviously, there is a limit to this improvement. A person with an average V_{O_2} (2.5 l. oxygen/min.) cannot, under any exercise regimen, attain the V_{O_2} (6 l. oxygen/min.) required of Olympic competition in endurance events.[2]

Regularity and Progression. Sporadic or infrequent exercise will not enhance physical fitness. It can even be detrimental to persons in whom fitness mechanisms have adapted to decreased metabolic demands or when the performer is in ill health.

The consensus of experts is that physical fitness can be developed through participation in three to five 30-minute exercise bouts per week.[1,8,18] One should be skeptical of the many commercial programs that are purported to cause miraculous fitness gains through several minutes of non-strenuous exercise per day.

The duration and intensity of exercise should be substantially below full capacity when commencing a fitness program, and should be increased gradually as fitness improvements are evidenced. An adult who desires to enhance endurance for muscular work could aim at upgrading overload to a maximal level at which he is capable of sustaining 20- to 30-minute exercise bouts at a heart rate of about 200 less his age in years. However, he should initiate the program with shorter periods of exercise that push heart rate no more than 120 to 140 beats per minute. Every two to four weeks the duration of the exercise bout could be lengthened by several minutes, and the task intensified to a degree where heart rate increases 10 heart beats per minute above the previous level.

Regression in performance and some local muscle-joint soreness and stiffness are often experienced during initial stages of exercise as the body adapts to newly imposed demands.[1] Fitness improvements may not be felt for several weeks to a month. Exhaustion, as evidenced by severe muscle pain, general body discomfort, and nausea during or following exercise, reflects too intense an overload or incomplete recovery from the previous exercise bout.

THE EXERCISE BOUT

A 5- to 10-minute preparation period called a *warm-up* should always precede stressful exercise. Jogging, light intensity calisthenics, and sport skills performed at a reduced pace are popular warm-up tasks. Warm-up readies the performer physiologically as well as psychologically for the more intense demands that follow. The increase in body temperature lessens muscle viscosity. The nerve impulse is believed to travel faster at higher temperatures making for improved neuromotor control when body heat is elevated.[2] The muscle capillaries dilate and the heart rate is raised gradually, thus better preparing the O_2 transport system for the increased cellular demands of exercise. Athletes have long known that proper warm-up leads to improved muscular work and motor performance levels. A *cool-down* or tapering-off period consisting of light activity such as jogging, and deep breathing aids the elimination of lactic acid, facilitates recovery of fitness organs, and provides for dissipation of body heat following strenuous physical activity.

TRADITIONAL CALISTHENIC WARM-UP EXERCISES

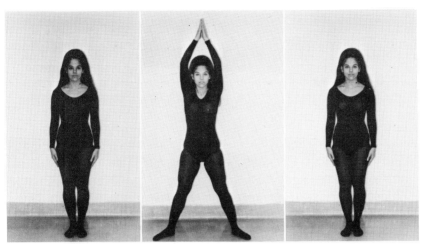

1. Jumping Jack
Stand with feet together, arms at sides. Jump so legs are apart, arms extended over head. Jump back to starting position.

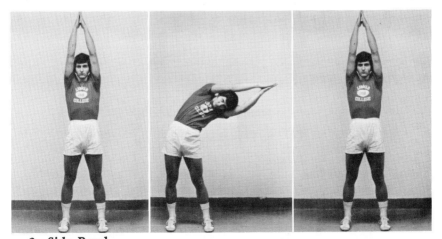

2. Side Bend
Stand with feet shoulder-width apart, arms extended overhead. Bend from waist toward the left without twisting body or lifting feet from floor. Return to starting position. Repeat toward right.

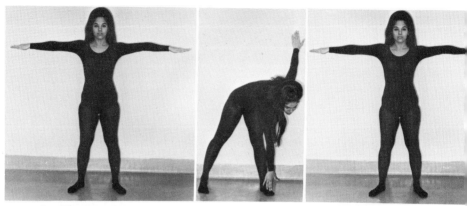

3. Hip Rotation and Toe Touch

Stand with feet about 2 feet apart, arms raised shoulder height, at sides, elbows fully extended, palms facing downward.   Twist toward left and touch toes of left foot with right hand, keeping knees straight. Return to starting position.   Repeat toward right side.

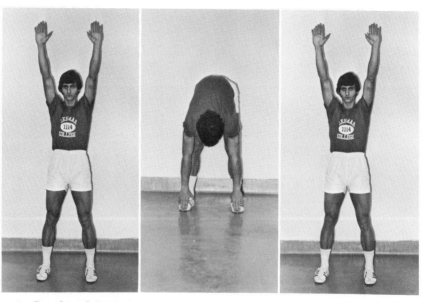

4. Bend and Stretch

Stand with feet shoulder-width apart, arms extended over head. Bend forward from waist and touch toes with hands without bending knees. Return to starting position.

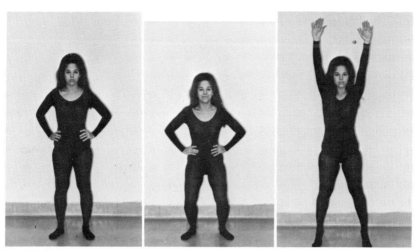

5. Half Squat and Stretch

Stand with feet shoulder-width apart, hands on hips. Keep back straight and feet flat on floor. Lower body by bending knees. Return to starting position and rise up off heels, arms extended over head. Return to starting position.

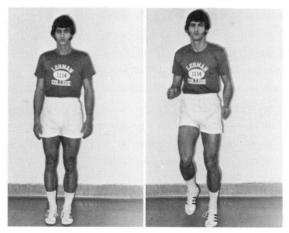

6. Jog in Place

Stand with feet together, arms at sides. Alternate raising feet about 6 inches from floor by bringing knees toward hips. Allow arms, bent at elbow, to swing forward and backward naturally.

EXERCISE PRECAUTIONS AND RECOMMENDATIONS

Body heat can be produced at a rate 10 to 20 times the resting level during stressful muscular work. The blood transfers this heat to the skin where it is given off to the air through sweating. The excessive loss of fluids resulting from intensified sweating could lead to a deficiency of body water. Muscle cramps, heat exhaustion, and even heat stroke are potential consequences of the inability to lose body heat to the environment.

The intensity and duration of exercise should be curtailed during initial exposure to a warm or high humidity atmosphere, especially if in an unconditioned state. Continuous exposure to heat (or cold) causes a gradual acclimation and improved temperature stress tolerance. Year-round training also enhances physiological adjustments to heat. Drinking water, juices, and other fluids prior to, during, and after exercise offsets loss of fluids through sweating. There is little need for ingestion of salt tablets unless one engages daily in long periods of highly intense exercise. Salt lost during exercise within a normal range is usually replaced by the diet. Clothing that provides freedom of motion and allows for maximum loss of body heat should be worn. Shorts, swimsuits, perforated shirts, and any material allowing exposure of limbs and loose enough to permit the circulation of air over the skin are recommended. When exercising in a cold environment loosen clothing during work performance and cover body parts during inactivity.

Stressful muscular activity following the ingestion of large quantities of drink and food disturbs digestion and limits performance. Sometimes a *stitch*, which is a pain felt in the side above the hip, possibly caused by a lack of oxygen to respiratory muscles, forces an individual to rest or reduce his exercise intensity. *Second wind* is the subsidence, when a steady state is reached, of the discomfort and rapid breathing experienced at the outset of strenuous exercise. Proper warm-up and the avoidance of heavy eating prior to exercise should promote second wind and reduce the chances of developing a stitch.

POTENTIAL PHYSIOLOGICAL EFFECTS OF EXERCISE

Research has produced common findings about the physiological effects of exercise. It should be realized that the morphological and functional adaptations to exercise are influenced by the constitutional characteristics and health habits of the participant. Certainly the outstanding fitness levels of great runners and swimmers are highly dependent on physiological advantages that are endowed, as well as by diet, sleep, relaxation, and other positive health variables.

Endurance exercise increases volume, hemoglobin, and erythrocytes of the blood, and lowers high blood pressure to a more normal level.[8] Blood vessels seem to maintain elasticity and suppleness when stressed systematically. Probably the most beneficial exercise effect is to the heart. The combination of a more forceful systole and a lengthening of diastole results in the ability of the heart to pump a larger volume of blood per beat. During exercise the heart should be capable of producing an increased cardiac output with a lower cardiac cost. The heightened cardiac output is evidenced by a greater heart rate reserve for more stressful exercise. The work of the heart could decline by as much as 72,000 foot-pounds per day through a more efficient cardiac output.[8]

Endurance exercise causes an increase in breathing depth and a decrease in the rate of breathing. A larger portion of the lungs open to air and blood flow. The overall operational efficiency of the respiratory muscles is improved. Less oxygen is demanded and blood flow to them is reduced, allowing a larger volume of blood to be supplied to activated muscle tissue. Thus, the work of breathing for high intensity muscular work is lessened. Reduction in cardiac cost and a quicker recovery for all intensities of muscular work reflect an improved degree of functioning by the O_2 transport system.

TABLE 5.1
Summary of the Effects of Training on Organs and Organ Functions*

	Increase	Decrease
A. Neuromuscular-Skeletal Effects		
1. Strength of bones and ligaments	X	
2. Thickness of articular cartilage	X	
3. Muscle mass (hypertrophy)	X	
4. Muscle strength	X	
5. Muscle elements—ATP, CP, myoglobin, K^+	X	
6. Muscle capillary density	X	
B. Cardiovascular Effects		
1. Blood volume and hemoglobin	X	
2. Maximal cardiac output	X	
3. Stroke volume (rest, submaximal & maximal)	X	
4. Oxygen consumption in maximal work	X	
5. Maximal blood lactic acid	X	
6. Resting heart rate		X
7. Heart rate during submaximal work		X
C. Respiratory Effects		
1. Maximal pulmonary ventilation	X	
2. Diffusion capacity in maximal work	X	
D. Other Changes		
1. Muscular work capacity	X	
2. Specific gravity of body	X	
3. Adipose tissue (body fat)		X
4. Serum triglycerides		X

* Adapted from Astrand and Rodahl, *Textbook of Work Physiology*, New York: McGraw-Hill Book Co., 1970, pp. 378–380. (Used with the permission of McGraw-Hill Book Company.) These changes have resulted in controlled experimental studies.

Progressive overload produces growth of muscle cells and connective tissues within joints and muscles as well as local vascularization. The magnified blood supply enhances muscle-joint endurance. Improvements in muscle endurance combined with beneficial adaptations in O_2 transport mechanisms have resulted in increases of 10 to 20% in oxygen consumption and 38% in oxygen debt tolerance.[8,4] The growth of intramuscular and intrajoint tissues causes hypertrophy and improved resiliency of muscles, tendons, and ligaments. The muscle grows in strength and the joints are better able to withstand the shock and stress of movement. Often overlooked is the potential influence of exercise in bringing about a rearrangement of the internal cellular structure of bones giving them added strength.

As related in Chapter Two, exercise combined with a slight curtailment in food intake can produce an increase in the specific gravity of the body and a decrease in skinfold thickness, reflecting a reduction of body fat.[2] Reductions in fat will lower metabolic costs of activities as well as stresses to heart and blood vessels. In sum, regular exercise can contribute to a more favorable body composition, greater movement efficiency, and heightened capacities for aerobic and anaerobic work.

REFERENCES

1. Adams, William C., et al. *Foundations of Physical Activity.* Champaign, Ill.: Stipes Publishing Company, 1968.
2. Astrand, O., and K. Rodahl. *Textbook of Work Physiology.* New York: McGraw-Hill Book Co., 1970.
3. Amussen, E. The Neuromuscular System and Exercise. In H. B. Falls (Editor), *Exercise Physiology.* New York: The Academic Press, 1968.
4. Andersen, K. L. The Cardiovascular System in Exercise. In H. B. Falls (Editor), *Exercise Physiology.* New York: The Academic Press, 1968.
5. Brouha, L. Training. In W. Johnson (Editor), *Science and Medicine in Exercise and Sports.* New York: Harper & Row, Publishers, 1960.
6. Cooper, Kenneth H. *Aerobics.* New York: M. Evans and Co., 1968.
7. Corbin, Charles B., et al. *Concepts and Experiments in Physical Education.* Dubuque, Iowa: Wm. C. Brown Co., Publishers, 1968.
8. deVries, Herbert A. *Physiology of Exercise for Physical Education and Athletics.* Dubuque, Iowa: Wm. C. Brown Co., Publishers, 1966.
9. Golding, L. A., and R. R. Bos. *Scientific Foundations of Physical Fitness Programs.* Minneapolis: Burgess Publishing Company, 1967.
10. Gutin, B. Pre-Season Conditioning. *The Athletic Journal,* 49:58–59, 1968.
11. Johnson, Perry B., et al. *Physical Education: A Problem-Solving Approach to Health and Fitness.* New York: Holt, Rinehart & Winston, 1966.
12. Margaria, R., and P. Cartelli. The Respiratory System and Exercise. In H. B. Falls (Editor), *Exercise Physiology.* New York: The Academic Press, 1968.
13. Mateeff, D. Problems of the Fight for Longevity. *Quest,* III, 41–50, 1964.
14. Mathews, D., and E. Fox. *The Physiological Basis of Physical Education and Athletics.* Philadelphia: W. B. Saunders Co., 1971.
15. Rasch, Philip. *Weight Training.* Dubuque, Iowa: Wm. C. Brown Co., Publishers, 1966.
16. Ricci, Benjamin. *Physical and Physiological Conditioning for Men.* Dubuque, Iowa: Wm. C. Brown Co., Publishers, 1966.
17. Sorani, Robert. *Circuit Training.* Dubuque, Iowa: Wm. C. Brown Co., Publishers, 1966.
18. Updyke, W., and P. Johnson. *Principles of Modern Physical Education, Health, and Recreation.* New York: Holt, Rinehart, & Winston, 1970.

CHAPTER SIX

Individualized Exercise
for Men and Women

Reading is to the mind what exercise is to the body.
RICHARD STEELE

EXERCISE FOR THE FEMALE

One need only observe women athletes to know that the majority of them possess grace and femininity. There is no scientific basis for the stereotyped mesomorphic body build associated with women who exercise. Because they are subject to the same biological laws, women and men can meet similar physiological needs through exercise. Physicians report that mild to vigorous physical activity ameliorates painful menstruation. Evidently demanding activities involving jumping, twisting, stretching, and jarring should be avoided during the first two days of the menstrual period, when the womb is quite heavy and engorged with blood. Submaximal exercise during the rest of menstruation is completely safe. Heavy exercise does not seem to affect the onset of menarche.

Regular exercise may aid childbearing and birth. Medical research indicates that female athletes are less subject to uterine disorders, have a shortened duration of labor, and have fewer complications while giving birth than do nonathletes.[4] Moderate rather than stressful muscular work activity is advocated for pregnant women.

Some teenage girls and women have exercise capacities superior to certain males. Yet, the female in general falls below the male in anaerobic and aerobic powers due to the basic structural and functional differences between the sexes. The maximal V_{O_2} of women is on the average 70 to 75% that of men.[1] Females are usually shorter and weigh less than males. The musculature of a man constitutes a greater percentage of his body weight, whereas women have about 10% more adipose tissue than do men. Thus, they may

61

be better able to withstand cold because of thicker, subcutaneous fat layers, but their strength level for any muscle group is about two thirds that of men.[1] This morphological difference between the sexes may also be a prime reason that the metabolic rate of a female is 6 to 10% lower than that of a male of comparable size.[4]

The heart, lungs, and thoracic cavity of a woman are often smaller than a man's. A most pronounced difference between the sexes is the female's smaller stroke volume and higher heart rate during exercise.[1] Females have fewer erythrocytes and less hemoglobin than do males because of their smaller blood volume.

EXERCISE PROGRAMS

It is beyond the scope and purpose of this book to discuss all existing exercise programs. Other references may be consulted if such information is desired. The four general categories of exercise described can be individualized for development and maintenance of optimal physical fitness.

Sport. Regular participation in swimming, tennis, skiing, handball, squash, basketball, volleyball, soccer, and the like can contribute to the efficiency of the O_2 transport system, muscle-joint endurance, and a favorable energy balance. Physical fitness benefits are determined in accordance with physiological demands. As these requirements of the sport bout are increased, aerobic and anaerobic powers are taxed more. If sport is to be an effective physical fitness tool there should be a progressive increase in the intensity, duration, and number of sport bouts performed per week. In this manner physiological demands are heightened gradually along with the body's capacity to meet them. The reader could consult Dr. Kenneth Cooper's *The New Aerobics*[2] for a detailed explanation and listing of sport fitness programs.

Jogging. Jogging is probably the most elementary, inexpensive, and personally geared exercise program known. Gross muscle groups and ankle and knee joints are taxed by jogging, and heart rate can be raised and

TABLE 6.1
Walk-Jog-Run Exercise Program for Men and Women

		Intensity Level		
	Time (*min.*)	Low	Middle	High
Warm-up	9	Walk briskly	Walk-jog	Jog
Body	15	Walk-jog	Jog	Jog-run
Cool-down	6	Walk briskly	Walk-jog	Jog

held at a critical threshold level. An example of a walk-jog-run program for men and women is presented in Table 6.1. This exercise program has built-in warm-up and cool-down and can be started at three different levels of intensity depending on fitness. Overload, when desired, is easily incorporated by traveling a longer distance during the 15-minute exercise bout.

Weight Training. Exercise with traditional weights, barbells, or dumbbells is better suited for muscle-joint development than any other type of activity. A core of four to eight exercises varying in *sets* (the number of times the core is repeated) and *repetitions* (the number of times each exercise is performed during a set) is usually included in weight training programs (Table 6.2). Progressive overload is applied by increasing the load ($2\frac{1}{2}$ pounds for women and 5 pounds for men) when 10 repetitions can be performed for each set.* The program would be initiated with resistances that are one fourth to one half the maximum strength capacity for that muscle group (see Laboratory Four, pp. 131–133). A program designed more for strength than endurance would involve fewer repetitions and greater loads

TABLE 6.2
Weight Training Prescription*

Exercise Set	Load Resistance	Repetitions
1	$\frac{1}{2}$ full load	10
2	$\frac{3}{4}$ full load	10
3	Full load	10

* From *Physical and Physiological Conditioning for Men* by Benjamin Ricci, copyright © 1966 by Wm. C. Brown Co., Publishers. Used with the permission of Wm. C. Brown Co., Publishers.

* In lifting a weight or other heavy object from the floor, spread feet for balance and stability, keep head up, and spine straight. Lower body to the object by bending knees and lift by straightening legs.

WEIGHT TRAINING EXERCISES

Body Area	*Exercises*
Upper Extremity	1 to 7
Lower Extremity	8 to 10

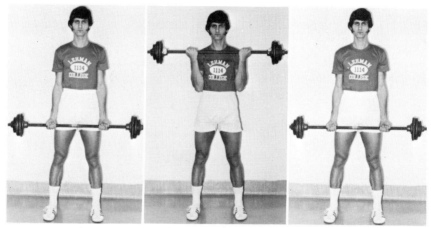

1. Arm Curl

Stand with feet shoulder-width apart. Grasp bar with hands turned inward and arms straight, elbows close to sides. Keep back straight and bring bar toward chest by flexing elbows. Return slowly to starting position. (Can also be performed with one arm using a dumbbell.)

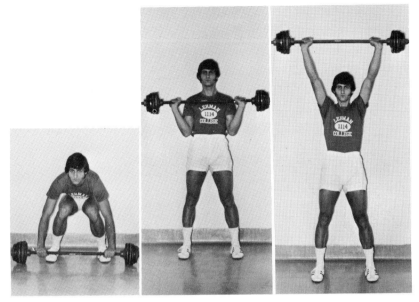

2. Press

Stand with feet shoulder-width apart. Turn hands outward to grasp bar and bring bar to front of chest. Keep legs and back straight as bar is pushed over the head by extending elbows. Lower gradually to starting position. (Can also be done in supine [lying on back] position on floor or bench.)

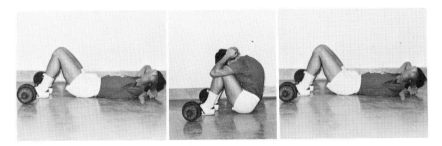

3. Sit-Up

Lie on back with knees bent, feet flat on floor. Take weight and hold behind head. Curl head and chest slowly so that lower back is off floor. Return to starting position. (Can be made more intense by performing movement on an inclined board.)

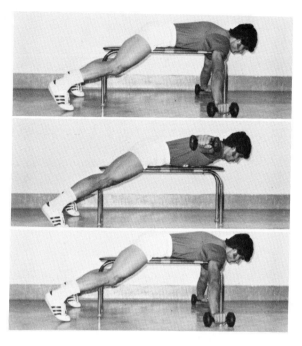

4. Prone Lateral Raise

Lie on stomach on a bench with legs spread to sides, feet on floor. Let arms hang straight down from shoulders and grasp dumbbells with hands turned outward. Raise arms to side to shoulder height with elbows extended. Return to starting position.

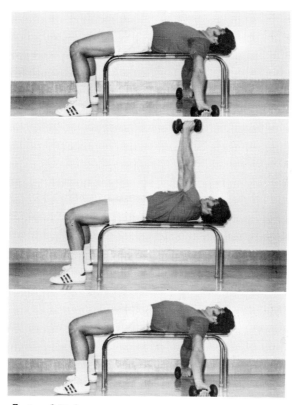

5. Supine Lateral Raise

Lie on back on a bench with legs spread, feet on floor. Grasp dumbbells with hands turned inward and raise arms to side to shoulder height with elbows extended. Draw straightened arms up and over chest and bring them together. Return to starting position.

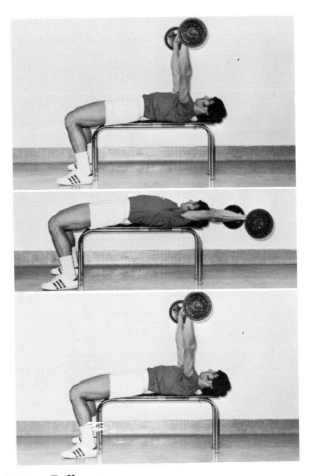

6. Straight Arm Pullover

Lie on back on a bench with legs spread, feet flat on floor. Grasp bar with hands turned outward and hold directly over chest with arms straight. Lower bar slowly to a position over the head keeping elbows extended. Return to starting position.

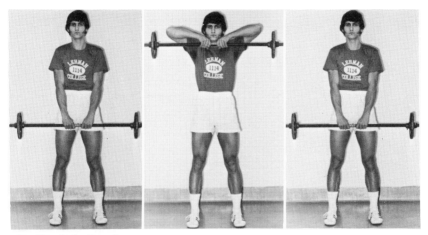

7. Upright Rowing

Stand and grasp bar with hands turned outward and about 4 inches apart. Hold bar directly in front of body with arms straight. Pull bar up by bringing hands just below chin keeping elbows above hands. Return to starting position.

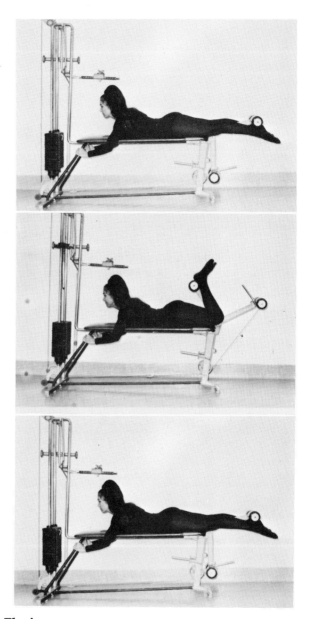

8. Knee Flexion

Lie on stomach on a work bench or table with legs straight and feet together. Draw heels to back of thighs by bending knees. Return slowly to starting position. Resistance can also be applied manually or with a weighted boot. This exercise can be performed with one or both knees.

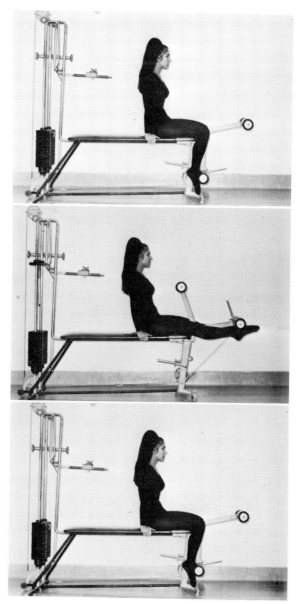

9. Knee Extension

Sit at the edge of a work bench or table with knees bent and legs dangling. Extend knees to a locked position, keeping back straight. Return slowly to starting position. Resistance can also be applied manually or with a weighted boot. This exercise can be performed with one or both knees.

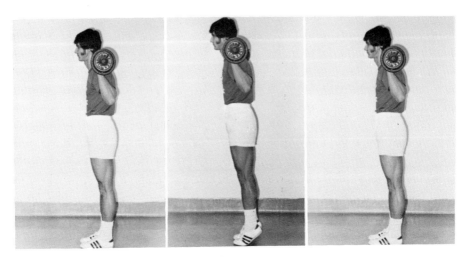

10. Ankle Extension

Stand and hold bar behind neck and on top of shoulders. Spread feet about 8 inches apart. Rise off heels keeping legs and back straight. Return to starting position.

Circuit Training.   Circuit training, in addition to stressing muscles and joints, places demands on the O_2 transport system, because exercise is performed within a set period of time.   Circuits have been prescribed (Royal Canadian 12 Minute X B X Plan for Women and the 11 Minute 5 B X Circuit for Men[9]) or they can be self-constructed. The major circuit variables are the *target time*, the time allotted to complete the exercise bout, and the circuit load.   The *circuit exercises*, which are the activities performed in sequence for three sets and the repetitions of each exercise per set, constitute the circuit load.

The selection of circuit and weight training tasks depends on specific muscle and joint weaknesses.   Exercises for the neck, shoulders, arms, chest, back, mid-section, legs, and ankles are included in a general circuit or weight training program.   They should be performed through full range of joint action to promote muscular development as well as joint flexibility.

To establish circuit time and load, as many repetitions as possible for each circuit exercise are performed in set time ranging from 30 to 60 seconds. A two-minute rest is taken between each exercise test.   Upon completion of the testing, the circuit is constructed by recording one half to three fourths the repetitions performed for each circuit exercise within the test period. Circuit target time is calculated by adding the testing times for each circuit exercise and multiplying by three.   Table 6.3 presents a circuit devised through this methodology.   The three sets of the circuit exercises are to be

TABLE 6.3
Circuit Training Exercise Program

Circuit Exercise	Testing Time (seconds)	Maximum Repetitions	Fractions	Circuit Repetitions
Jumping jacks	60	60	$\frac{3}{4}$	45
Push-ups	30	15	$\frac{1}{2}$	8
Sit-ups	60	30	$\frac{1}{2}$	15
Squat-thrusts	60	45	$\frac{1}{2}$	23
Step-ups	60	32	$\frac{3}{4}$	24

Total Testing Time = 4:30 × 3 = 13:30 Circuit Time

completed without a rest. The first set should be accomplished quite easily, because it is subminimal muscular work. Overload takes effect during the later stages of the second set and throughout the third set when the performer approaches a maximum or nearly maximum exercise load. Progressive overload can be applied by decreasing the circuit time, increasing circuit exercise repetitions, or performing exercises with weight resistance.

CALISTHENIC EXERCISES FOR CIRCUIT TRAINING*

Body Area	Exercises
Abdomen	1 to 4
Back	5 to 8
Sides of the Waist and Buttocks	9 to 12
Hips and Legs	13 to 15
Wrist, Arms, and Chest	16 to 19

* Exercises progress from light to heavy intensity for each body area.

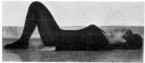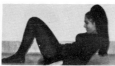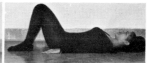

1. Head and Shoulder Raise
Lie on back with knees bent, feet flat on floor close to buttocks, arms at sides. Curl head, shoulders, and upper back off floor. Return to starting position.

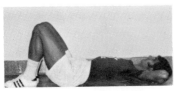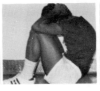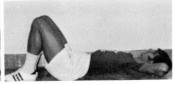

2. Bent Knee Sit-Up

Lie on back with knees bent, feet flat on floor, close to buttocks. Clasp hands behind head. Curl head and shoulders and proceed to raise back completely off floor. Return to starting postion.

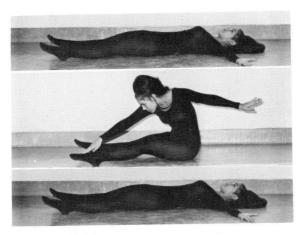

3. Sit-Up and Toe Touch

Lie on back with legs straight, feet spread about 2 feet apart. Extend arms at side to shoulder height. Curl head, shoulders, and back off floor and toward the left touching left toe with right hand. Return to starting position and repeat toward right side.

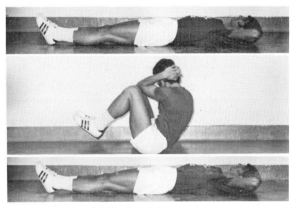

4. Bent Knee Sit-Up and Hip Rotation

Lie on back with legs straight, hands clasped behind head. Draw both knees upward and curl upper body off floor. Twist toward the right and touch right knee with left elbow. Return to starting position and repeat toward the left side.

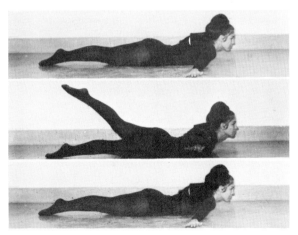

5. Single Leg Raise

Lie on stomach with legs straight, feet together, arms raised at sides to shoulder height, elbows fully extended. Slowly raise left leg about 2 feet off floor keeping knee extended. Lower slowly to starting position. Repeat with right leg.

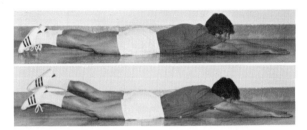

6. Flutter Kick
Lie on stomach with legs straight, feet together, arms extended over head. Raise both legs about a foot off floor keeping knees extended. Alternately whip legs up and down.

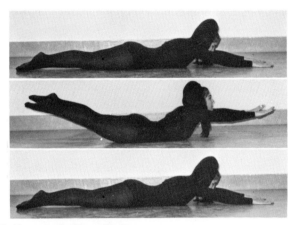

7. Double Leg and Chest Raise
Lie on stomach with legs straight, feet together, arms extended over head. Raise chest and outstretched arms as high off floor as possible while doing the same with legs, keeping knees extended. Hold for five seconds and return to starting position.

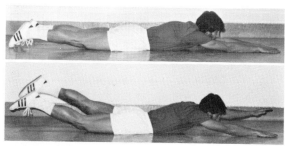

8. Arm and Leg Flutter

Lie on stomach with legs straight, feet together, arms extended over head. Raise chest and outstretched arms as high off floor as possible while doing same with legs, keeping knees extended. Alternately whip arms and legs up and down.

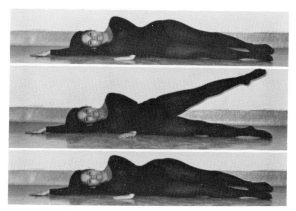

9. Single Leg Raise Sideways

Lie on right side with head resting on right arm which is extended over head. Bend left arm and brace left hand against floor in front of chest. Keep legs straight with left leg on top of right leg. Lift left leg upward until it forms a 30° angle with the floor. Lower leg to starting position.

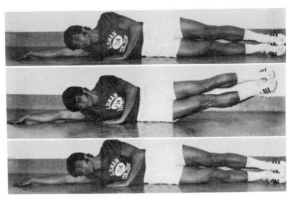

10. Double Leg Raise Sideways

Lie on right side with head resting on right arm which is extended over head. Bend left arm and brace left hand against floor in front of chest. Keep legs straight with left leg on top of right leg. Slowly raise both legs from the floor as high as possible and lower slowly.

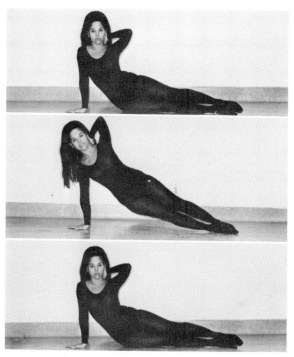

11. Side Trunk Raise

Lie on right side with right hip, leg and foot on floor. Keep left leg
on top of right leg. Hold right arm straight to support upper body
which is raised off floor. Clasp left hand behind neck. Raise hips as
far off floor as possible, hold for about five seconds, return to starting
position.

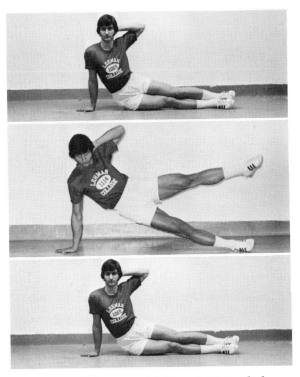

12. Single Leg Raise Sideways with Trunk Extended

Lie on right side with right hip, leg, and foot on floor. Keep left leg on top of right leg. Hold right arm straight to support upper body which is raised off floor. Clasp left hand behind neck. Raise hips as far as possible off floor and lift left leg upward as far as possible, keeping knee extended. Lower leg and hip to floor.

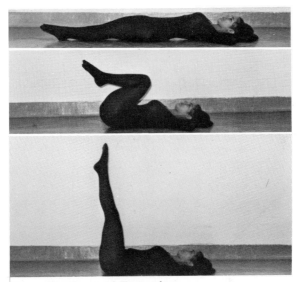

13. Double Knee Flexion and Extension

Lie on back with legs straight, feet together, hands clasped under head. Keep back straight and draw knees toward chest. Straighten legs upward without lifting hips. Lower legs slowly to starting position by reversing the pattern.

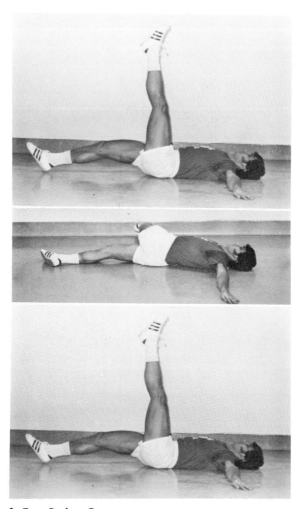

14. Single Leg Swing Over

Lie on back with left leg raised straight upward, right leg on floor. Raise arms to shoulder height. Swing left leg across body until left foot touches floor. Return to starting position. Repeat with right leg.

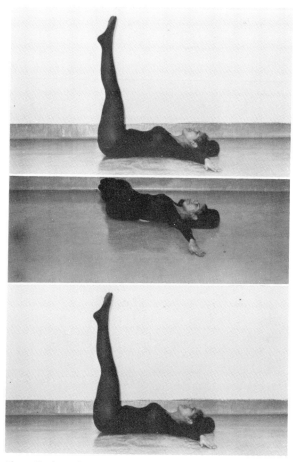

15. Double Leg Swing Over

Lie on back with both legs raised straight upward. Raise arms at sides to shoulder height. Swing both legs across body toward left side and touch floor with feet. Return to starting position. Repeat toward opposite side.

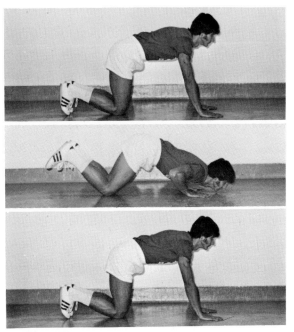

16. Kneeling Push-Up

Kneel with arms straight, hands on floor directly below shoulders. Raise feet off floor about 4 inches and lower chest to floor, keeping back straight.   Slowly push up to starting position by extending elbows.

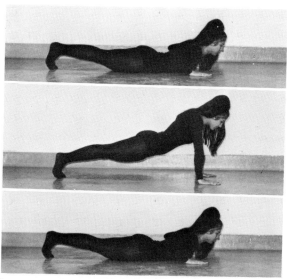

17. Push-Up

Lie on stomach with legs straight, feet together. Bend arms and place hands on floor next to shoulders. Push up by extending elbows, keeping upper body and legs in a straight line. Return slowly to starting position.

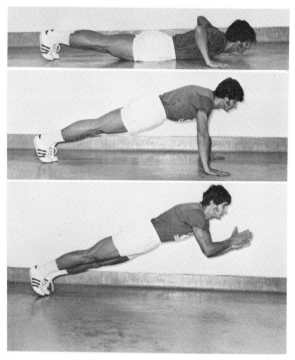

18. Extended Arm Push-Up

Lie on stomach with legs straight, feet together. Bend arms and place hands on floor about 5 inches to sides of shoulders. Push up by extending elbows, keeping upper body and legs in a straight line. Return slowly to starting position. To make this exercise more intense, push up with greater power and clap hands together before returning to starting position.

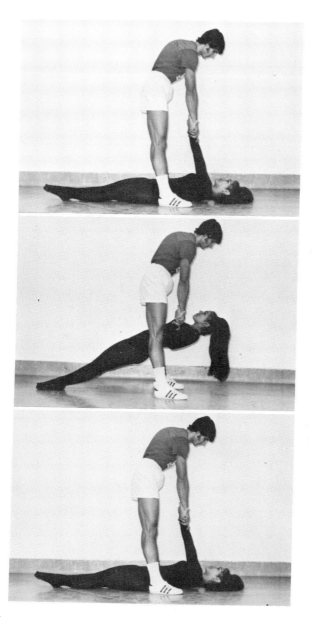

19. Chin

Lie on back between the legs of a partner who stands. Clasp wrists of partner with elbows fully extended. Slowly raise upper body by bending elbows to 90° angle, keeping a straight line from shoulders through hips. Hold for two seconds and return slowly to starting position. Can also be performed from traditional chinning bar.

SELECTION OF INDIVIDUALIZED EXERCISE

The kind and amount of exercise should be determined with care at any stage in life. Exercise should be individualized, that is, geared to sex, needs, capacities, and interests. The practicality of the exercise should also be considered because it is almost impossible to participate faithfully in an activity that is too expensive, time-consuming, or unrewarding in terms of providing some measure of satisfaction.

The suitability of exercise depends in part on metabolic requirements, which are determined by the nature of the movements involved, the manner in which they are performed, the duration of the exercise bout, and the physiological condition of the performer. The caloric consumption per minute for handball is approximately five times greater than for golf. However, golf or some other intermittent exercise activity might very well be a suitable task for a person who had been ill or bedridden for a long period of time. In fact, a completely sedentary person should increase heart rate no more than 30 to 40 beats per minute above the resting level when commencing an exercise program.

Exercise should have carry-over value so that it can be continued throughout life. Actually there is little need for commercial fitness plans involving elaborate facilities, because the quality of the performance is more crucial to beneficial physical fitness outcomes than is the area used. Fitness development through sport can be time-consuming. It has been estimated that a one-hour bout of handball or basketball would be necessary to stress the aerobic processes of the body to the same degree as running a mile in six minutes and thirty seconds.[2] Sport performance can be expensive when costly equipment and fees for use of facilities are required. Adequate skill and knowledge are also requisite to regular participation in sports. Yet, sports reward participants a high degree of satisfaction and have a great potential for systematic engagement throughout life.

In terms of accessibility, it is much easier to organize play for sports such as tennis, handball, and two-man basketball than for football, soccer, softball, and other team sports that necessitate the recruitment of other players.

Sports are inherently dangerous. Muscle strength and joint stability often prevent or limit the severity of injuries that can be caused by the stresses and strains of sports. When a person engages in tennis, skiing, handball, or other strenuous sports once a week or every other week, the muscles, joints, and O_2 transport system may never become conditioned to meeting the demands of the activity. Dry mouth, nausesa, and respiratory difficulties sometimes accompany the activity and the aftereffects of fatigue such as muscle pain and general body tiredness may be experienced. Several jogging, circuit, or weight training bouts each week using the joints and muscle groups stressed can aid the individual to handle the physiological requirements of sport and to reap better performances as an athlete.

Jogging, circuit training, and weight training are better systematized and controlled than are sport fitness programs. Overload also is more easily regulated and these programs have better built-in evaluation systems which provide feedback of how the performer is progressing. Most significant of all, fitness benefits are attained more readily because the exercise stress can be made more specific to the development of the quality desired. When a desired fitness level is achieved a sport probably is a good fitness maintenance exercise.

Jogging and circuit training require the least equipment and can be performed by groups or individually in almost any indoor or outdoor facility (playground, backyard, cellar, rooftop, garage, classroom, hallway, or corridor).

The initial exercise bouts in any exercise program are the most difficult and challenging. Persevere, enjoy them, overload gradually, and you will experience results. Once attained less effort is required to maintain a certain fitness level than to develop it. Progressive overload can cease. However, strenuous physical activity must be continued regularly. Physiological changes produced by overload are temporary, and the body will eventually revert back to its original state if systematic exercise of sufficient intensity and duration is discontinued completely. Exercise for pleasure does not necessitate adherence to a strict program of set activities. Flexibility and variations in exercise schedules are refreshing and desirable.

REFERENCES

1. Astrand, O., and K. Rodahl. *Textbook of Work Physiology*. New York: McGraw-Hill Book Co., 1970.
2. Cooper, Kenneth H. *The New Aerobics*. New York: M. Evans and Co., 1970.
3. Cooper, Kenneth H. Quantifying Physical Activity—How and Why. Proceedings of the National Workshop on Exercise in the Prevention, in the Evaluation, and in the Treatment of Heart Disease. (Supplement to *the Journal of the South Carolina Medical Association*), December, 1969.
4. Klafs, Carl, and D. Arnheim. *Modern Principles of Athletic Training*. St. Louis: The C. V. Mosby Company, 1969.
5. Maver, Jane A., et al. *Introduction to Human Movement*. Reading, Mass.: Addison-Wesley Publishing Co., 1968.
6. Rasch, Philip. *Weight Training*. Dubuque, Iowa: Wm. C. Brown Co., Publishers, 1966.
7. Ricci, Benjamin. *Physical and Physiological Conditioning for Men*. Dubuque, Iowa: Wm. C. Brown Co., Publishers, 1966.
8. Sorani, Robert. *Circuit Training*. Dubuque, Iowa: Wm. C. Brown Co., Publishers, 1966.
9. Royal Canadian Air Force. Exercise Plans for Physical Fitness. *This Week Magazine*, Mount Vernon, N.Y., 1962.

CHAPTER SEVEN

Exercise and Health

Most Western Nations are increasingly afflicted by a variety of pathological conditions, collectively designated as "hypokinetic diseases," which are attributable in a major or minor degree to the generally prevailing lack of exercise. These diseases, disorders, aches and pains concern chiefly the muscular and cardiovascular systems, metabolism and emotional patterns. They cause a premature reduction of earning power, early invalidism, and widespread mortality from functional and degenerative cardiovascular derangements.

Hans Kraus, M.D.
AND
Wilhelm Raab, M.D.

CORONARY HEART DISEASE

Coronary heart disease (CHD) is the general term for the forms of heart disease associated with narrowing, occlusion, or bursting of the coronary blood vessels.

The tragedy so typical of coronary heart disease struck the Stilwell family of San Francisco, California, one summer evening. George Stilwell, head of the household and successful business executive, suffered ventricular fibrillation—a common form of heart attack. He was rushed to the hospital, but died leaving his wife with four fatherless children. That he died of heart disease is not unusual, because approximately 700,000 Americans have had similar fates each year for the past 20 years. What does make the Stilwell case relevant is the fact that he was a jogger, who ran a mile course about three times a week for three years prior to his death. Like others in sedentary occupations, this middle-aged man felt a need for a regular routine of vigorous exercise, and he chose jogging. Not only did he jog, but he recorded his times with a stopwatch, ever hoping to improve his previous performance. On the evening he died, Stilwell attempted to go the mile in six minutes, a feat he had not accomplished in the past.   Unfortunately, the combination of a late heavy lunch still being digested, the stresses of a busy day, and the strenuous exercise placed too much strain on his heart.[10]

The reality of a person dying, or even being disabled, as a result of physical activity provides ammunition for skeptics who question the values of exercise. It might be concluded that the Stilwell case lends support to the contention that moderate or strenuous exercise can be damaging to a *healthy* heart. However, it would be erroneous to assume a cause-effect relationship here between the exercise bout and the heart disease.   The postmortem examination revealed that Stilwell's three major coronary arteries had been badly impaired by thick layers of fatty deposits.   In fact, one of the arteries was completely blocked. It was obvious that the buildup had been taking place for years.

Autopsy studies show that young men and women, even teenagers, have the beginnings of atherosclerosis, the narrowing of coronary blood vessels. When the condition is not ameliorated the deterioration can continue slowly and steadily, eventually culminating in a heart attack in later years.   Each winter in the northern areas of the country instances are reported of persons who suffer heart attacks as a result of shoveling snow.   There is a tendency to implicate the shoveling of snow as the sole cause of the heart attack.   Shoveling snow, jogging, and other physiological or psychological stressors are really catalysts that induce the final and most devastating phase of a disease that probably existed for an extensive time period.   According to current morbidity and mortality statistics millions of American men and women might be progressing toward the fatal stages of coronary heart disease in the absence of overt symptoms.

Few effective diagnostic tests or devices measure cardiovascular health directly.   The electrocardiogram (ECG) commonly utilized by physicians does not always reveal signs of coronary heart disease.   An objective indicator of the functioning of the cardiovascular system now being incorporated into medical examinations is the response of the heart to muscular work demands.   Chest pain, discomfort, abnormal elevations in heart rate, and slow recovery of heart rate to resting level following moderate exercise may be symptomatic of cardiovascular inadequacies.   The mortality from heart disease in Swedish males, 35 to 44 years of age, is about one quarter that of their American counterparts.[4]   The fact that Swedes have higher maximal oxygen consumption levels at younger ages lends support to the contention that a high capacity for exercise might be a reflection of cardiovascular health.

Laboratory studies by exercise physiologists show (for specific populations) that systematic exercise of sufficient intensity produces increments in cardiac output, maximal oxygen consumption, blood volume, and blood hemoglobin (see Chapter Five).   It would be desirable to ascertain if these training effects are accompanied by a reduction of susceptibility to heart attack.   Epidemiological studies have been conducted in the United States, Europe, and Israel since 1950 to test the hypothesis that the greater the amount of exercise performed regularly, the smaller the risk of developing coronary heart disease.[6,9,16,21] The major criterion for exercise in most of these studies has been occupation. Thus, bus drivers, clerks, and subjects in other sedentary jobs have been compared to peers involved in higher energy expenditure occupations. A consistent finding is that those participating in occupations involving moderate exercise have better prospects, statistically speaking, of both avoiding and delaying coronary heart disease than do persons in sedentary jobs.

An investigation reported in the British journal *Lancet* represents the initial attempt to test the hypothesis that "vigorous" leisure-time exercise, intense enough to produce a "training" effect, will lower the incidence of coronary heart disease.[15] In this study 16,882 male office workers aged 40 to 64 from across Britain were the subjects. They recorded all their daily activities for Friday and Saturday over the course of two years from 1968 to 1970. These activities were analyzed and those likely to cause a peak energy output of 7.5 kcal. per minute were classified as vigorous. The rationale was that high intensity exercise taken in short bouts (a minimum of 30 minutes) would involve more than 50% maximal oxygen consumption, and thus increase cardiac output substantially. It was assumed that functional changes in the cardiovascular system were not likely to occur with steady state exercise of longer duration. Over the two-year period 232 of the subjects suffered a first clinical heart attack. Each subject of a heart attack was matched with two colleagues not so affected. Eleven percent of those developing coronary heart disease compared to 26% of the controls reported participation in vigorous exercise. Thus, habitual vigorous exercise during leisure time seemed to reduce the incidence of heart attack in middle-aged sedentary men. The researchers concluded: "Training of the heart and cardiovascular system is *one* of the mechanisms of protection against common risk factors and the disease (CHD)."[15]

There were obvious weaknesses and limitations in this British study as well as in others conducted prior to it. The study depended on a questionnaire, that is, the subjects reported their exercise patterns. The definition of "vigorous" exercise used in the study could be far stricter. Evidently, the physiological requirements of exercise depend on three major variables: (1) the nature of the exercise activity, (2) the manner in which it is performed, and (3) the physiological condition of the performer. Thus, because of variances in the latter two variables, the range of energy expenditure for any reported exercise bout could be quite wide. The investigators themselves admit that: "how often men in their sixties—or for that matter their forties—actually reached peaks of 7.5 kcal. per minute during their exercise activities, we do not know."[15] With the exception of cigarette smoking, investigators did not explore the potential influence of other hereditary, personality, and life style variables on the onset of coronary heart disease.

Even when attempts are made, it is difficult to control such variables. For example, it is quite natural for subjects to constantly vary their living habits. Changes in any significant mode of life could elicit a CHD response that might be attributed invalidly to exercise, or to the lack of it.

Despite the facts that exercise can produce favorable functional cardiovascular changes, and that studies show the incidence of heart attacks to be higher in sedentary subjects than in active ones, it would be premature to regard exercise *alone* as a panacea for heart disease. The consensus of authorities is that coronary heart disease is associated with a set of risk factors including: (1) sex, (2) family history, (3) diet, (4) cigarette smoking, (5) high blood pressure, (6) high levels of blood fats, (7) heart beat irregularities, (8) lack of exercise, and (9) personality. (Dr. Friedman is convinced that the great majority of heart disease victims show the same common traits of excessive ambition, overwhelming aggression, impatience, and slavishness to the clock [Type A personality]. The more relaxed, easy-going Type B personality is less prone to heart attack.[10]) The determination of the relative contribution of each of the risk factors as well as their mode of interaction remains to be ascertained.

George Stilwell made the greatest omission of his life by failing to seek relevant feedback from proper professionals to appraise his coronary risk factors. Vigorous exercise without a prior medical examination and consultation with a physician eventually proved disastrous to himself and his family. Heart attack candidates, like Stilwell, can take constructive action to offset all risk factors other than those relating to family background. In fact, the only preventive measure against coronary heart disease available to twentieth-century man is to reduce the potential influence of as many of these coronary risks as possible.

Proper exercise seems to implement the recovery of heart attack patients, as well as others bedridden for extensive time periods. Prolonged rest in the horizontal position incapacitates cardiovascular efficiency, reduces muscle tone, and impairs renal functioning.[17] Prior to the 1940s hospital patients who remained in bed for weeks had difficulty in regaining body stamina. Heart attack victims often suffered heart failure upon rising, because the heart was incapable of adapting to the sudden stress of standing. Today it is quite common for surgical and coronary patients to participate in graded programs of suitable exercise as soon as possible during their recovery process.

The limited study to date seems to indicate that *hypertension* (high blood pressure) appears less frequently and at later stages in life in physically active persons than sedentary ones, and that systematic exercise can produce favorable adaptations to certain respiratory diseases such as emphysema.[18] Yet, it would be premature to state conclusively that exercise will either reduce the severity of these disorders or enhance recovery from them.

OBESITY AND BLOOD LIPIDS

The avoidance of excess body fat is a constructive health measure that is often ignored in practice. The enlargment of visceral organs, such as the kidney and liver, respiratory and circulatory difficulties, high accumulations of carbon dioxide in the blood, and the increased risk of suffering atherosclerosis, hypertension, diabetes, gallstones, and coronary heart disease are related to being obese. Obesity complicates and adds to the severity of angina, varicose veins, bone and joint disorders, and predisposes the individual to bodily injury resulting from the incapacity to withstand the stresses of movement. Study confirms that reduction of fat to normal levels is often followed by a temporary remission of overt diabetes.[18] Common problems in pregnancy and difficulties in giving birth, directly associated with obesity, accentuate the significance of maintaining a lean body mass by women.

Reproach and ostracism of the obese can result in psychological difficulties, especially in the young when an awareness of the opposite sex develops, and the need for compassion, love, and understanding is crucial to the molding of a mature, healthy personality. Thus, although not a disease in itself, obesity is definitely a twentieth-century health problem of the first magnitude. The relevance of systematic exercise to health is reaffirmed when one considers its contribution to control of obesity (see Chapter Two).

Exercise seems to have several potential beneficial effects on the metabolism of *cholesterol* and *triglyceride*, the major blood fats. Since the triglyceride molecule can be broken down for fuel consumption, exercise can inhibit and reduce its concentration in the blood.[18] Blood lipids are related positively to percentage of body fat. If body fat is reduced, blood fat concentration may also be lowered.

LOW BACK PAIN

According to Kraus and Raab underexercise can result in muscular weakness, tightness, and tension that often lead to postural defects or localized muscular pain, especially in the lower back.[11] From a study conducted by them 80% of all back difficulties were found to be muscular in origin. They also contend that nervous tension contributes to localized muscle-joint pain. Exercise fosters muscle strength and endurance as well as joint stability and can serve as an outlet for nervous tension. Thus exercise can be a critical variable in the prevention of and recovery from low back pain and other neuromuscular disorders. Over the course of eight years, pain and stiffness in the lower back suffered by 233 patients subsided with gains in strength and flexibility produced by systematic exercise, and relapsed when exercise was discontinued.[11]

AGING

There is no adequate proof that regular exercise will either add or subtract years from one's life. However, it appears that exercise can impede some of the natural biological changes that the body undergoes as it grows older chronologically (Table 7.1). Physically active persons seem to maintain their muscular work capacity and the functional and structural processes

TABLE 7.1
Summary of Physiological Changes in Aging

	Decrease	Increase
A. O$_2$ Transport System		
1. Lungs		
Compliance in lung tissue and chest wall	X	
Alveolar volume	X	
Vital capacity (after age 30)	X	
Pulmonary ventilation	X	
2. Heart		
Maximal Vo$_2$	X	
Systolic blood pressure and mean arterial pulse pressure		X
Maximal heart rate	X	
Heart weight and heart volume		X
B. Neuromuscular System		
Muscle strength	X	
C. Other Changes		
Heat tolerance	X	
Return of body temperature to normal following heat exposure	X	
Tendency to suffer heat stroke		X
Body weight		X
Percentage of body fat		X
Work capacity	X	

associated with it longer. Such persons can be considered "physiologically younger" than sedentary ones of the same age who have lower muscular work abilities.

Professor Nicholas Testa, a colleague of mine, is a perfect example of a 44-year-old man who literally possesses the body of a much younger man. When polio struck him earlier in life he proceeded to recondition atrophied muscle groups through extensive daily exercise, which has since remained an integral part of his life. Presently Professor Testa is capable of jogging $2\frac{1}{4}$ miles in less than 15 minutes, and in one-minute periods can perform over 55 sit-ups, 45 squat jumps, and 20 chins. In our human performance laboratory we estimated his percentage of body fat to be 9, well below the level indicative of obesity. For two years in succession he has won the physical fitness intramural at Lehman College, competing against the most fit male college students approximately 20 years younger than himself.

In sum, most authorities agree that individualized exercise, along with proper sleep, nutrition, and relaxation, is a constructive health measure. It would be wise for men and women of all ages to exercise regularly, but they should do so sensibly in order to enjoy it and make themselves feel better.

REFERENCES

1. American Heart Association. *So More Will Live. A Report to the American People.* New York Times, Section II, January 29, 1967.
2. Astrand, O., and K. Rodahl. *Textbook of Work Physiology.* New York: McGraw-Hill Book Co., 1970.
3. Burt, John J. Cardiovascular Health. *Journal of Health, Physical Education and Recreation,* 32:36-37, 1968.
4. Cooper, Kenneth H. Quantifying Physical Activity—How and Why. Proceedings of the National Workshop on Exercise in the Prevention, in the Evaluation, and in the Treatment of Heart Disease. (Supplement to the *Journal of the South Carolina Medical Association*), December, 1969.
5. deVries, Herbert A. *Physiology of Exercise for Physical Education and Athletics.* Dubuque, Iowa: Wm. C. Brown Co., Publishers, 1966.
6. Gilmore, C. P. The Real Villain in Heart Disease. *New York Times Magazine,* March 25, 1973.
7. Hoyman, Howard S. Our Modern Concept of Health. In J. H. Humphrey, et al. (Editors), *Readings in Health Education.* Dubuque, Iowa: Wm. C. Brown Co., Publishers, 1964.
8. Ismail, A. H. Body Composition and Relationships to Physical Activity. In H. B. Falls (Editor), *Exercise Physiology.* New York: The Academic Press, 1968.
9. Jenkins, Robert. Implications of Current Physiological Research to Physical Education. *New York State Journal of Health, Physical Education and Recreation,* 20:26-31, 1968.
10. Kiester, Edwin. Your Personality Can Be a Matter of Life or Death. *Today's Health,* 51:16-19, 1973.
11. Kraus, Hans, and Wilhelm Raab. *Hypokinetic Disease.* Springfield, Ill.: Charles C Thomas, Publisher, 1961.
12. Life-Time Inc. *The Healthy Life.* New York: Time, Inc., 1966.
13. Mayer, Jean. The Best Diet is Exercise. *The New York Times Magazine,* April 25, 1965.
14. Mayer, Jean. *Overweight.* Englewood Cliffs, N.J.: Prentice-Hall, Inc., 1968.
15. Morris, J. N., et al. Vigorous Exercise in Leisure Time and the Incidence of Coronary Heart Disease. *Lancet,* 1:333-339, 1973.
16. Raab, W. Prevention of Degenerative Heart Disease by Physical Activity. *Quest,* III:19-30, 1964.
17. Ryan, A. J. The Physician and Exercise Physiology. In H. B. Falls (Editor), *Exercise Physiology.* New York: The Academic Press, 1968.
18. Skinner, James S. Longevity, General Health, and Exercise. In H. B. Falls (Editor), *Exercise Physiology.* New York: The Academic Press, 1968.
19. Updyke, Wynn F., and Perry Johnson. *Principles of Modern Physical Education, Health, and Recreation.* New York: Holt, Rinehart & Winston, 1970.
20. White, P. D. An Ounce of Prevention. *New York Times Section II,* January 29, 1967.
21. Exercise: Does It Help Ward Off Heart Trouble? *Consumer Reports,* 32:141-145, 1968.

Index

Laboratory Workbook

Name _____ Section _____ Date _____

LABORATORY ONE

Muscular Work Capacity

There are innumerable kinds of muscular work. Environmental and individual variables influencing work capacity differ from one situation to another. As Astrand stated:[1] "It is impossible to present one formula that takes into account all aspects of man's maximal work capacity, since the demands set by different types of activities vary greatly."

The *Step Test*[4] and *12-Minute Run Test* are objective measures of the capacity to perform specific types of muscular work. Both tests are quite practical in that they do not involve intricate equipment.

The performer must be in excellent medical condition and should engage in three to six exercise sessions prior to attempting these or other tests of physical fitness. Heavy exercise by a completely sedentary person will most likely produce severe muscle soreness and other symptoms of fatigue. If severe chest pain or breathing difficulty is experienced while being tested, stop immediately.

A. CALCULATING HEART RATE

Place tips of middle and index fingers on carotid artery of the neck which is under the jaw next to the Adam's apple. Press in *lightly* until the pulse is felt. Count the number of pulse beats for 60 seconds, 30 seconds (multiply by two), and 15 seconds (multiply by four). Have two other testers do the same. Record results below.

HEART RATE DATA

Method	Self	Tester 1	Tester 2
1 minute			
30 seconds × 2			
15 seconds × 4			

B. THE MODIFIED STEP TEST FOR MEN AND WOMEN

Subjects work in pairs. A leader or instructor keeps the step-up cadence through use of a metronome set at 120. (A watch may be used to keep count if there is no metronome available.) Subject steps up and down a 16- to 17-inch high bench at the rate of one complete step every two seconds, or 30 steps per minute. A step consists of going up with the left foot and the right foot, then coming down with the left foot and the right foot. Men continue the task for *three* minutes; women for *two* minutes. Partner should make sure subject maintains cadence. Stop exactly when supposed to, sit down, and remain still. After one minute partner takes subject's heart rate for a 30-second period. Multiply count by two.

Using norms below, evaluate your performance and record results.

STEP TEST NORMS[4]

Rating	Men	Women
Poor	Above 125	Above 135
Average	111–124	121–134
Above average	100–110	110–120
Excellent	Below 100	Below 110

Date	Heart Rate	Step Test Rating

C. THE 12-MINUTE WALK-RUN FOR MEN AND WOMEN

The subject walks/runs as far as possible during a 12-minute period. The greater the distance of the run the better the test score will be. It is recommended that a steady pace be maintained for the 12 minutes.

The test may be performed on a regulation running track marked at 25-yard intervals, or a 100-yard straightaway divided by 25-yard markers as diagrammed below. Subjects work in pairs; one counts laps (each 100 yards), the other runs. The instructor tells the performers the amount of time that has elapsed.

X   Instructor

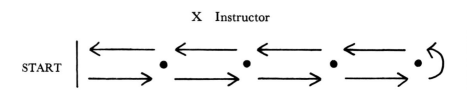

START

Calculate the distance traveled to the nearest 25-yard marker. Using the norms below, evaluate your performance and record results.

12-MINUTE RUN TEST NORMS[3]

Distance in Miles		Performance Rating
Male	Female	
1.86	1.5	Excellent
1.82	1.4	Very good
1.74	1.3	Above average
1.61	1.2	Average
1.58	1.1	Below average
1.52	1.0	Poor
1.48	0.9	Very poor

Date	Distance	Performance Rating

Questions

1. Did your performances on the Step Test and 12-Minute Run Test correspond?
2. How would you evaluate your muscular work capacity?
3. Explain what these ratings might signify in terms of physical fitness.

Name _____ Section _____ Date _____

LABORATORY TWO

Body Weight

The purpose of this laboratory is to determine the degree of obesity or thinness, and to demonstrate the potential of a caloric imbalance in creating a weight problem.

A. DETERMINATION OF PERCENT OF BODY FAT BY SKINFOLD MEASURES

Each subject measures and records the various skinfold measures listed below (see page 18 for directions). To ensure reliability, three measures are obtained and the average used to predict percent of body fat and specific density.

Skinfold	Measurements in Millimeters			
	1	2	3	Average
Women: *Iliac crest* (just above the pelvis in the middle of the body at the side)				
Triceps (back of the upper arm between the top of the shoulder and the elbow)				
Men: *Triceps* (see above)				
Chest (just above and to the right of the right nipple)				
Abdominal (just to the right of the navel)				

From the average measures above, determine the percent of body fat and specific density from the nomograms for men and women on pages 106–107. Record below.

    A. Specific gravity prediction _____

    B. Percentage of body fat   _____

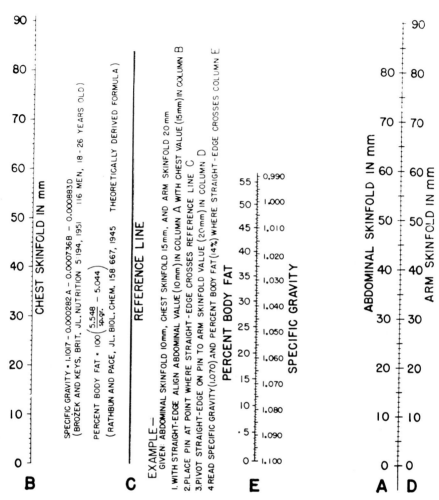

Nomogram for conversion of skinfold thickness to specific gravity in young men. (From *Physiological Measurements of Metabolic Functions in Man* by Consolazio, Johnson and Pecora, copyright 1963. Used with permission of McGraw-Hill Book Company.)

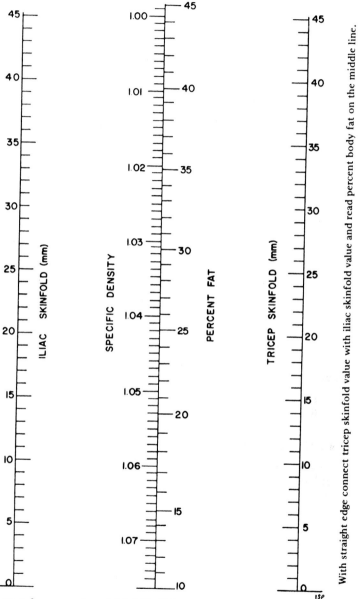

Nomogram for conversion of skinfold thickness to specific gravity in young women. (From *Concepts in Physical Education: With Laboratories and Experiments* by Corbin, Dowell, Lindsey and Tolson, copyright 1970. Used with permission of Wm. C. Brown Company Publishers.)

Using the norms below, evaluate percent of body fat.

BODY FAT NORMS*

Classification	Men (%)	Women (%)
Excellent	0– 6.3	0– 8.0
Very good	6.4– 7.2	8.1–11.0
Above average	7.3– 9.0	11.1–14.0
Average	9.1–12.2	14.1–17.0
Below average	12.3–13.1	17.1–19.0
Poor	13.2–19.9	19.1–24.0
Very poor	20+	25+

* From *Concepts in Physical Education: With Laboratories and Experiments* by C. Corbin et al., copyright © 1970 by Wm. C. Brown Co., Publishers. Used with permission of Wm. C. Brown Co., Publishers.

B. COMPARISON OF BODY WEIGHT TO IDEAL WEIGHT

Record height and weight below. Stand facing away from the scale with heels together, dressed in gym uniform or underclothes (no shoes). Compress the hair with the stadiometer and read on the scale to 0.5 inch. Record weight to the largest whole pound.

      A. Weight   ————————————

      B. Height   ————————————

Determine ideal weight by consulting height-weight tables on page 19.

      A. Ideal weight range   ————————————

      B. Calculated weight   ————————————

C. SUBJECTIVE EVALUATION OF BODY TYPE

Stand in front of a full-length mirror in gym uniform (men, no shirt). Study your back, front, and profile views. Rate endomorphic, mesomorphic, and ectomorphic characteristics of body according to a scale ranging from 7 to 1. (The more characteristics evidenced, the higher the rating.) Have your instructor and a classmate rate your body type. Record below and compare ratings.

BODY TYPE

Rater	Endomorph	Mesomorph	Ectomorph
Self			
Instructor			
Classmate			

D. DEGREE OF OBESITY OR THINNESS

From the information attained, circle the appropriate number along the continuum below.

Excessively lean		Lean		Average		Obese		Excessively obese
0	1 2	3	4	5 6	7 8	9		10

Questions

1. Are you overweight or underweight? By how many pounds?
2. What is your predicted specific density and percent of body fat?
3. What is your numerical body-type classification?
4. Does it appear that percent of body fat correlates with height-weight and body-type measures?
5. Explain why one might expect discrepancies among the measures attained, and why percent of body fat is the most significant indicator of body composition.

E. DETERMINATION OF CALORIC BALANCE

Ann Smith is a 5'5", 120-lb. college student. Her food intake and activity schedule for one day are given below. Calculate her total caloric intake and caloric output.

Meal	Food Intake	Calories Consumed
Breakfast:	1 glass orange juice	120
	2 strips bacon	81
	2 fried eggs	110
	1 glass milk	166
	1½ slices buttered bread	200
Lunch:	hamburger	350
	French fries (20 pieces)	275
	8 oz. cold	107
Dinner:	lettuce salad	32
	salad dressing—1 tablespoon	59
	3 oz. roast beef	189
	1 cup mashed potatoes	240
	1 cup broccoli	44
	1 cup diced carrots	44
	1 plain muffin	134
	1 glass milk	166
Snack:	¾ cup ice cream	205

CALORIC EXPENDITURE*

Activity	Hours	Calories Expended
Sleeping	8	
Sitting, reading	2	
Sitting, eating	1.5	
Sitting, writing	1	
Classwork, lecture	3	
Conversing	1	
Walking on level	1.5	
Standing, light activity	4	
Sitting, normal	2	

* Refer to the caloric expenditure table on pages 22 and 23 to determine expenditure for activities listed above.

Questions

1. What is Ann's total caloric intake?
2. What is Ann's total caloric expenditure?
3. What kind of caloric balance does Ann have on this particular day? By how many calories?
4. Barring other variables, if the same caloric imbalance occurred three times a week how many pounds could Ann gain in one year? (Calculate to nearest $\frac{1}{2}$ pound. 3,500 Cal. = 1 lb.)

Name _____ Section _____ Date _____

LABORATORY THREE

Effectiveness of the O₂ Transport System

This laboratory is designed to determine how efficiently heart, blood vessels, and lungs perform at rest and during muscular activity. It must be remembered that environmental and personal factors affect heart rate (HR). Thus, heart rate readings will vary from one observation to another. To assure reliable results during the following procedures, heart rate must be determined with care and precision. External and psychological factors should be controlled to avoid their contaminating effects. To obtain heart rate count pulse for 30 seconds and multiply by two.

A. EVALUATION OF RESTING HEART RATE

Sit relaxed for three minutes and then take heart rate for three trials. Take average and circle your average heart rate on the scale below.

Trial	Heart Rate
1	
2	
3	
Average heart rate	

RESTING HEART RATE SCALE[3]

45 – – 50 – – 55 – – 60 – – 65 – – 70 – – 75 – – 80 – – 85 – – 90 – – 95

Excellent	Good	Average	Poor

B. HEART RATE CHANGES IN DIFFERENT POSTURAL POSITIONS

Record heart rate for each of the following activities. Maintain each activity for three minutes, and record on the bar graph below.

Activity	Heart Rate
Sitting	
Lying with feet elevated	
Standing at attention	
Slow walk	

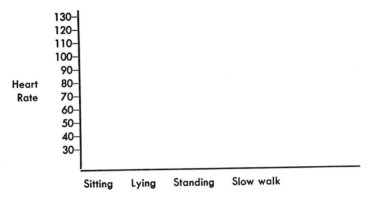

Heart Rate

130—
120—
110—
100—
90—
80—
70—
60—
50—
40—
30—

Sitting   Lying   Standing   Slow walk

Questions

1. Why does heart rate seem to increase as one changes from a lying to standing position?
2. Why does heart rate remain the same or decrease when one goes from standing at attention to a slow walk?
3. Why should one continue to exercise lightly (rather than sit or lie down) following strenuous exercise?
4. How can one rest the heart?

C. CARDIAC COST (CC) AND RECOVERY FROM WORK

Take heart rate following each work task and at one-minute intervals for five minutes.

Work Intensity (Step-Up Task)*	Time	Post-activity	1 Min.	2 Min.	3 Min.	4 Min.	5 Min.
Light	30 sec.						
Moderate	2 min.						
Heavy	5 min.						

* Thirty steps per minute on a 12- to 20-inch high bench. Subjects may be unable to maintain 30 steps per minute. They should attempt to keep pace as best they can. Substitute running in place if there is no access to benches.

Record information from above table on the following graph. Use different types of lines to represent each exercise task.

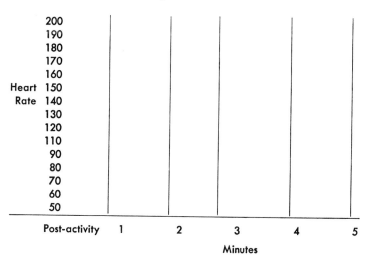

On the graph below plot your heart rates for *heavy* exercise along with heart rates of the person in the class who came closest to full cardiac recovery after five minutes of rest.

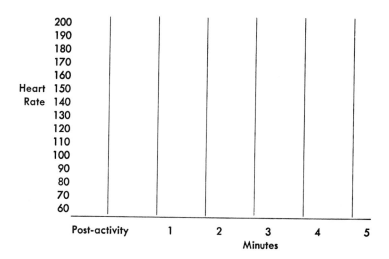

Questions

1. How do your recovery rates for post-heavy exercise compare with quickest rates?
2. Subjectively evaluate your O_2 transport system.

Name _____ Section _____ Date _____

LABORATORY FOUR

Joint-Muscle Identification and
Strength-Endurance Evaluation

This laboratory involves the identification of the joint action and muscle used in popular movement activities and an evaluation of strength-endurance of major muscle groups.

A. JOINT ACTION AND MUSCLE IDENTIFICATION

Determine the joint, joint action, and agonist used in the activities listed below.

Activity	Joint	Joint Action	Agonist
Calisthenic Exercise 1. Head rotation			
2. Chin			
3. Push-up			
4. Sit-up (knees bent)			
5. Half squat			
6. Lying lateral single leg raise			
7. Flutter kick from prone position			
8. Heel raise			
Weight Training Exercise 1. Press			
2. Arm curl			
3. Straight arm pullover			
4. Double knee extension			
5. Double knee flexion			
6. Ankle extension			

Combined Movements

1. Jumping jack	1. Shoulder	1	1
		2	2
	2. Hip	1	1
		2	2
2. Football punt (lower extremity)	1. Hip	1	1
	2. Knee	2	2
	3. Ankle	3	3

B. ISOTONIC STRENGTH AND ENDURANCE OF MAJOR MUSCLES*

Calculate the weight in pounds for each of the exercises listed below by taking the recommended percentage of total body weight. Slowly perform as many repetitions as you can for each exercise through full range of movement. Use the scale below to rate muscle strength-endurance capacity for each exercise.

Body weight_____lb.

RATING SCALE

Repetitions		Rating
Male	Female	
Less than 3	Less than 2	Very poor
4	3	Poor
5–8	4–7	Fair
9–11	8–10	Good
12–16	11–14	Very good
More than 17	More than 14	Excellent

* For health and safety reasons, students should engage in neuromuscular training on three to five occasions prior to actual testing. Weight training is slowly becoming an accepted activity for girls and women, and they can engage in this exercise for evaluation purposes.

Exercise	% Body Weight	Lb.	Reps.	Rating
Double arm curl	One-third			
Bench press	Two-thirds			
Lateral pull down	Two-thirds			
Upright rowing	One-third			
Double knee extension	Two-thirds			
Double knee flexion	One-third			
Ankle extension (heel raise)	Body weight +40 lb.			
Sit-up	One-fifth			

Questions

1. Explain the steps involved in determining the joint action and muscle used in performing a specific movement.
2. What specific strength-endurance deficiencies are reflected in the data attained from Exercise B?

Name _____ Section _____ Date _____

LABORATORY FIVE

Individualized Exercise for Men and Women

The purpose of this laboratory is to participate regularly in individualized exercise programs and to evaluate such experiences in terms of effects and subjective feelings. It is also designed to demonstrate the potential role of exercise in weight control, and to aid in the sensible selection of physical activities for adult participation.

A. APPRAISAL OF INDIVIDUALIZED EXERCISE

Participate in jogging and either a weight *or* circuit training program. If desired and time permits, engage in both weight and circuit training. Exercise bouts are to be performed three to four times a week for five weeks* in each program.

Jogging. The walk-jog-run program outlined in Table 6.1, page 62, is to be utilized. The beginning intensity is based on the results of the 12-Minute Run Test (page 103); low intensity for those scoring poor, middle intensity for those in the fair to good range, and high intensity for those scoring in the excellent category. Distance traveled during the 15-minute body of each exercise bout is to be recorded below. Retake the 12-Minute Run Test after five weeks of rhythmic training.

_____

*Five weeks is probably the minimum time period in which physiological changes can be produced through systematic training.

Pre-12-Minute Run Test

Date_____ Distance_____ Rating_____

Week	Exercise Bout	Distance	Week	Exercise Bout	Distance
1	1		3	4	
	2				
	3				
	4		4	1	
				2	
2	1			3	
	2			4	
	3				
	4		5	1	
				2	
3	1			3	
	2			4	
	3				

Post-12-Minute Run Test

Date	Distance	Rating

Questions

1. Compare pre- and post-training performances for the 12-Minute Run Test.
2. Summarize your post-exercise feelings during the first and last week of walk-jog-run programs.

B. WEIGHT TRAINING

Select five or more weight training exercises (pages 64–72) for general development or for specific muscle-joint weaknesses (Laboratory Four). See Chapter Six, page 63, for recommended beginning resistances and weight training prescription. After five weeks repeat Exercise B, Laboratory Two.

WEIGHT TRAINING PROGRAM

Resistance (lb.)

Weight Training Exercise	Week 1	Week 2	Week 3	Week 4	Week 5

C. CIRCUIT TRAINING

Select five or more circuit training exercises (pages 73–87) for general development or specific muscle-joint weaknesses. See Chapter Six, page 72, for directions in creating the circuit. After five weeks repeat Exercise B, Laboratory Two.

CIRCUIT TRAINING PROGRAM

Circuit Exercise	Testing Time (sec.)	Maximum Reps.			Fraction	Circuit Reps.		
		Test 1	Test 2	Test 3		Test 1	Test 2	Test 3

Total time:_____

×3_____

Circuit target time:_____

CIRCUIT RECORD

Week	Exercise Bout	Circuit Target Time	Time to Complete Circuit
1	1		
	2		
	3		
	4		
2	1		
	2		
	3		
	4		
3	1		
	2		
	3		
	4		
4	1		
	2		
	3		
	4		
5	1		
	2		
	3		
	4		

Questions

1. What effects did the weight or circuit training have on muscular strength and endurance levels?
2. Summarize your post-exercise feelings following exercise work-outs during the first, third, and fifth week of training.

D. EXERCISE FOR OBESITY CONTROL

Assume that you have a constant weekly positive caloric balance of 350. Design two exercise programs to ward off creeping obesity. Incorporate three to five work-outs per week to magnify caloric expenditure and thus create a negative caloric balance. Utilize jogging in one program and a sport in the other. Refer to Table 2.2, pages 22 and 23, for expenditure figures for jogging and sports. Show calculations and record descriptive exercise information below.

Activity	Amount of Time/Period	Periods/Week	Total Calories Expended
Jogging			
Selected sport			

Calculations:

E. EXERCISE SELECTION

Rank the six activities in Table L-5.1 that produce the highest total point values (determined by adding the numbers in each column). Column numbers in Table L-5.1 relate to the following scales:

Physical Fitness and Carry-over Value

3	Good
1	Average
0	Poor

Interest

3	High
1	Moderate
0	Slight

These six activities are suitable for continued participation through adult years. Discretion should be used in the final selection of activity. Personal limitations and chances for success should also be considered. A high point value may be attained in an activity in which interest is only slight or moderate. Interest may be heightened through instruction that develops skill and knowledge in that activity.

Exercises Suitable for Future Participation

1._____
2._____
3._____
4._____
5._____
6._____

TABLE L-5.1
Point Values for Physical Activities

Activity	Physical Fitness Benefits	Carry-over Value	Interest*	Total Points
Badminton	1	3		
Basketball	3	1		
Bowling	0	3		
Circuit training	3	3		
Fencing	1	1		
Golf	0	3		
Gymnastics	3	1		
Handball	3	3		
Personal defense	1	1		
Jogging	3	3		
Skiing	3	3		
Soccer	3	0		
Softball	0	1		
Swimming	3	3		
Scuba diving	1	3		
Squash	3	3		
Tennis	2	3		
Touch football	1	1		
Track and field	3	1		
Volleyball	1	1		
Wrestling	3	0		
Weight training	3	3		

* Determine a point value for each activity based on interest.

REFERENCES

1. Astrand, O., and K. Rodahl. *Textbook of Work Physiology.* New York: McGraw-Hill Book Company, 1970.
2. Consolazio, C. F., et al. *Physical Measurements of Metabolic Functions in Man.* New York: McGraw-Hill Book Company, 1963.
3. Corbin, C. et al. *Concepts in Physical Education: With Laboratories and Experiments.* Dubuque, Iowa: Wm. C. Brown Co., Publishers, 1970.
4. Updyke, W., and P. Johnson. *Principles of Modern Physical Education, Health, and Recreation.* New York: Holt, Rinehart & Winston, 1970.